LOOK TEN YEARS YOUNGER

LIVE TEN YEARS LONGER

A MAN'S GUIDE

DR. DAVID RYBACK

PRENTICE HALL
Englewood Cliffs, New Jersey 07632

10   9   8   7   6   5   4   3   2   1

This book cannot and must not replace hands-on medical care or the
specific advice of your doctor. Use it instead to help you ask the right
questions, make the right choices, and work more closely with your
doctor and the other members of your health-care team.

Library of Congress Cataloging-in-Publication Data

Ryback, David.
  Look ten years younger, live ten years longer : a man's guide /
David Ryback.
     p.   cm.
  Includes index.
  ISBN 0–13–079344–2 (case). — ISBN 0–13–079336–1 (pbk.)
  1. Men—Health and hygiene.   2. Stress management.   3. Longevity.
I. Title.
RA777.8.R93   1995
613′.04234—dc20   95–34064
                                                                          CIP

ISBN 0-13-079344-2 (C)
ISBN 0-13-079336-1 (P)

PRENTICE HALL
Career and Personal Development
Englewood Cliffs, NJ 07632
A Simon & Schuster Company

PRINTED IN THE UNITED STATES OF AMERICA

CONTENTS

CHAPTER

1

GROWING OLD, STAYING YOUNG—1

CHAPTER

2

THINK YOUNG AND BE YOUNG—25

CHAPTER

3

ANTIAGING STRESS REDUCERS—49

CHAPTER

4

KEEPING YOUR SEXUALITY YOUNG AND STRONG—77

CHAPTER

5

THE MIDLIFE YEARS—115

CHAPTER

6

DR. RYBACK'S ANTIAGING FOOD PROGRAM—141

CHAPTER

7

EXERCISE AWAY THE YEARS—195

CHAPTER

8

KEEPING YOUR HEART STRONG—213

CHAPTER

9

AGE-PROOFING YOUR SKIN AND HAIR—235

CHAPTER

10

STOP SMOKING AND ADD YEARS TO YOUR LIFE—269

CHAPTER

11

AN EMPOWERED LIFESTYLE FOR LIVING LONGER—289

Clearly, if disease is man-made,
it can also be man-prevented.
It should be the function of medicine
to help people die young
as late in life as possible.

—Ernst Wudner

FOREWORD

As a physician and surgeon I can attest to the fact that we live in stressful times today. Drawing on his extensive experience, Dr. David Ryback has written a book all men can use to deal with this trying issue. As Dr. Ryback points out, stress can affect your health and even shorten your life, but only if *you* allow it to happen. Fortunately, there are many ways to control stress, reclaim your health, and even prolong your life span.

Thanks to TV and other mass media, today's world of short attention span bombards us daily with tons of information, much of it stressful and worrisome. Remote control in hand, we search for instant relief and gratification, fighting back against the ongoing blur of stressful sound bites.

Our personal, marital, and business relationships can be sources of stress as well, draining our energy and health. Between the covers of this revealing book can be found creative solutions to the stress we all feel, and ways to channel negative energy into positive and healthy pathways, even how to worry creatively and effectively.

Many of us men create our own stress because of what we have been taught about being successful. What we were not taught is that all of these ideals can take their toll on our health and enjoyment of life. What the author has done is to provide us with ways to discover such sources of stress and how to reverse their negative effects, while still achieving our goals and ideals.

At first glance, as you weigh this book in hand in search of a healthier mind and body, you might say, "This is too long a read. I want a quick answer to my problem and I don't have time to read all this." The fact is, you do not need to read the entire book—at first. The book is so well organized that you need only scan the chapter headings, find the section that deals with your problem, and find a number of options to correct that problem.

It appears that Dr. Ryback has left nothing out, covering all facets of mind and body, from both traditional and alternative viewpoints, to provide us with a choice of solutions. Books that offer one simple solution to life's complex problems often fail because one solution does not work for all men. Here, in this book, we find many possible solutions, whether our problems relate to aging, physical health, mental concerns, or the sexual arena, and we need use only what works best for our particular concerns.

While you need not read the entire book to find the answer to your specific problem, I would recommend keeping it at your bedside or wherever you relax. Read a little at a time, and you will learn creative ways to correct the many stressful problems you may have, both great and small.

The real value of this book, in my opinion, goes beyond looking younger and living longer. The bonus is that it can open doors to a better, more enjoyable life on a daily basis. What good is a longer life without higher quality? The bottom line is: If you feel good about yourself and enjoy your life with less stress, you will naturally and automatically look younger to everyone.

This book is a treasure chest of information and wisdom for all men. If you care about yourself at all, read this book! It will likely change your life, as it has mine.

Mark S. Davis, M.D.

INTRODUCTION

HOW THIS BOOK WILL HELP YOU LIVE LONGER

Suddenly as never before there is a national obsession with longevity, and men of the current Baby Boomer generation especially are courting longer life by focusing on virtually every facet of health and fitness. Scientists are discovering that people can live much longer than they have been, and census figures both reveal—and predict—this longer average lifespan. According to the Census Bureau, for example, the United States has at least 36,000 people over the age of 100. By the year 2020, there will be 266,000.

Two-thirds of Americans want to live to 100 years, according to a survey released by the Washington-based research group Alliance for Aging Research. Well, each of us can live to the age of 120, according to UCLA scientist Roy Walford. His theory is based on both his own hard data with those of Clive McKay in 1935. By minimizing calories, providing the correct nutrients and other measures, our lives can be extended quite significantly. But very few have done it—yet!

The average lifespan of men in the United States could be extended by 9.78 years, according to the American Heart Association, if deaths from heart disease alone could be eliminated. Imagine how your life expectancy could be extended if you went beyond having a healthier heart and also had a lean, fit body; less stress in your life; a healthier prostate gland; and a healthier attitude in general!

For the first time, a comprehensive approach to nutrition, fitness, and other aspects of health awareness makes the conservative promise of ten more youthful, healthy years of life. This book covers the most important of these lifestyle factors in a simple, yet personal manner. It cuts through the morass of overwhelming information and provides a coherent, straightforward series of suggestions targeted for the intelligent man who is willing to take the responsibility for living a longer, healthier, happier life.

Look Ten Years Younger, Live Ten Years Longer is an easy read backed by scientific research, that promises and delivers the information men need for ten more years of youthful life and appearance.

YOUR PERSONAL ROAD MAP TO LONGEVITY

Given the choice of just plain getting older or maturing youthfully, which would you prefer? Looking ten years younger and living ten years longer is definitely within your reach. Want to lose weight easily and permanently with little effort? Then read about the Ryback Food Plan and the importance of three-month cycles in losing weight for a lifetime. Want to acquire a fitness program that makes you sexier and increases your life span by at least ten percent? Read about the SPEAR approach and enjoy exercising for a more fit, muscular body. Want smoother, younger skin? Learn the natural path to a youthful look. Give up smoking when you're ready (despite multiple failings) by going through a four-step process and using the best quit-smoking technologies available. Learn brief, simple steps to deter cancer and give up chronic worry for peace of mind. Learn about getting the stress out of your life by making better choices and acting wisely so that you can live not only longer but more happily as well. And as you enjoy ten more years of a youthful life, learn how to "fine-tune" those extra years through specific suggestions for an active and satisfying sex life with your mate into and through the maturing years.

Never have men been more aware of nutrition, fitness, and general lifestyle enhancement. Some changes, such as avoiding obesity, quitting smoking, and preventing cancer are obvious. Others, such as learning your optimal dosage of vitamin C (different for each individual), reversing high blood pressure without medication, and understanding how having reliable support groups affects our aging process, are less obvious. This book explores each of these areas thoroughly, clearing up the confusion that many men feel.

All of us wish for extended youth and a longer life. Most of us would be willing to do what it takes to accomplish this if we had simple directions or guidelines that were (a) scientifically valid and (b) delivered in a credible style in (c) an easily read and understood format.

Look Ten Years Younger, Live Ten Years Longer appeals to those men who are interested in youth and life extension but have been disappointed by quick-fix remedies and scientifically unsound advice that fail in the end.

You've probably become cynical. You've heard of and tried many diets. You've seen Michael Landon go down with cancer, despite all attempts at "new age" cures. You're ready for some scientifically sound, simple truth: What really works, why, and how to do it in the most simple, direct way. This book serves that purpose.

A flurry of publications serves to illustrate a strong interest in the topic of longevity. There is ample evidence to support the contention that the desire for longevity is backed up by the research. *Look Ten Years Younger, Live Ten Years Longer* is clearly a book at the right time, offering you the benefits of practical advice plus scientific research, on how men can live ten years longer, and look ten years younger.

AVOID THE RAVAGES OF AGING

We start dying, statistically speaking, in our 60s and 70s, though scientists generally agree that our genetic makeup allows for a life of up to 110, and some even say up to 130 or 140 years. Yet to date very few of us have been reaching the age of 100.

How do we know when we're getting old, as opposed to maturing youthfully? Beyond the subjective perception, there are objective criteria: wrinkles in our skin give our age away; we forget what we used to remember effortlessly; we visit the doctor more frequently; we hear with increasing difficulty; we feel too tired to have fun with others; we become more cantankerous.

All these ominous indications of our mortality can be slowed down significantly and, in some cases, eliminated. We will all die eventually. But in the lives we do have, there is the opportunity to live longer and healthier, more sexually and joyfully, if we take the responsibility to do so.

And it's all so simple! Eat less, take your vitamins, do your exercise, take care of your skin, stay a step ahead of illness, and enjoy an ongoing, youthful attitude. So simple, at least in theory. The challenging part is to forge each of these elements into a lifelong pattern of habits; the sad truth is that because we don't follow through on these simple steps, one third of American men die of heart disease. One in four is stricken with some form of cancer which could be prevented in part by proper nutrition, good habits, and early detection.

I am confident that, by following through on my suggestions in this book, backed up by scientific research and consolidated to comprise a simple lifestyle approach, you can confidently anticipate ten more years of life—and look up to ten years younger than you do now, depending on how different your current lifestyle is from what you read in this book.

A PROMISE FOR LIFE IMPROVEMENT

I've spent the last few years researching the relevant literature and analyzing my own, as well as my patients', lifestyles. I've integrated this with my professional experiences lecturing in the United States, Canada, Europe and Asia, as well as with my own research findings.

In this book, I share with you the results of my efforts. You will learn not only how to acquire better eating habits and ways to change your values regarding physical fitness, but also how to make attitudinal and social changes that last, *and* become a greater lover. In many little ways, you will learn how to improve the quality of your life that will add up to a significant transformation.

Here is my promise: By opening this book, you've already taken the first step to becoming a healthier, more vital and more youthful individual. If you read, reread and follow through on my suggestions, within a three- to six-month period you will begin to notice a loss in weight, a feeling of greater vitality, and an improvement in the romantic and social aspects of your life, both at home and at work.

This is the first time all these factors have been combined in a single book that is based on sound research, yet remains a personalized and hopefully entertaining read.

SLOWING DOWN THE AGING PROCESS

Appearing 10 to 20 years younger than my age, I am living proof that this comprehensive approach works in my own life. No other book offers this combination of personal experience and scientific objectivity, of in-depth, practical advice with such a comprehensive range of health topics.

If you choose *not* to live your life in a healthful manner as the years go by, here's what will happen to the various systems in your body:

1. Your heart will become less efficient. Your arteries will become more rigid, less flexible; your blood pressure will begin to climb.

2. Your lungs will become less efficient as well. Volume will decrease and diffusion of oxygen across the membranes will be reduced.

3. Your brain will decrease in size—a 10 percent decrease between the ages of 30 and 70. The membranes surrounding your brain will begin to thicken. You won't see these changes directly, of course. What you will notice is a loss in short-term memory, a greater disposition to depression, and a more rigid outlook on life.

4. The bones of your skeleton will become thinner and weaker. Your vertebral disks may begin to deteriorate gradually, leaving you surprised one day when you discover that you're an inch or more shorter than the last time you were measured. Arthritis and other diseases of your bones and joints may become more prevalent.

5. Your muscles will become much weaker, and your coordination may suffer. Getting up from your chair will seem more of an effort.

The good news is that much of this can be either totally pre-vented or at least slowed down substantially. Through eating less, eating smarter, using the right regimen of supplements, exercising consistently and adopting the right attitude, as well as following through on the other recommendations of this book, you can stay healthier, look younger, and live longer. How much? Well, that depends on your genetic disposition, the present condition of your body, your degree of commitment, your present age, and where you live. To round it off to the most accurate number to cover the wide divergence among all readers, I feel very comfortable with the num-ber 10. For some men it may be more, for others less. But what's real-ly important is that by following through, you *will* be healthier, with stronger heart and lungs, a smarter, more responsive brain, a more attractive body, and more fulfilling relationships.

GROWING OLD, STAYING YOUNG

What better examples of growing old while staying young than Sean Connery and Paul Newman!

A popular newspaper survey found 64-year-old Sean Connery to be among the world's sexiest men, second only to Jean-Claude Van Damme. Among the top ten as well was 70-year-old Paul Newman. Such mature men as Connery and Newman can encourage the rest of us to take pride in our image, even through our 60s and 70s. As we live ten years longer, we *can* still look ten years younger. All it takes is a healthy approach to food, fitness, and attitude.

The potential for extending your life is now greater than ever. Although many of us have been brainwashed to believe that much of the physical deterioration associated with growing older is inevitable, this is clearly not so. Scientific proof, as well as my own experiences and those of my patients, provide convincing evidence that it *is* possible to stay younger while living longer.

In the early 1900s, people in their forties were considered old. By the 1930s, old age was considered to occur around the mid-sixties, thanks to gains in medicine, nutrition, and fitness. At present, life expectancy has grown to the early seventies for men and late seventies for women. By following the recommendations in this book, you can easily aspire to live into your eighties and even nineties.

SEVEN SECRETS OF ROBUST MATURE MEN

1. Take Care of the Body

Twenty years ago, young adulthood was considered to be between the ages of 18 and 22. A recent Gallup poll delivered the newly emerged range of young adulthood as between 18 and 40! We're definitely living longer and staying youthful for more extended periods. This quiet revolution of longevity means that as we live longer, we take on the responsibility of caring for a body that is pioneering a new path. Such courage deserves special consideration.

2. Continue to Expect Ongoing Energy and Endurance

We must learn to break tradition and destructive mythologies about aging. In terms of physical strength, we can continue to expect ongoing energy and endurance instead of settling into the proverbial rocking chair. At age 70 in 1984, Jack LaLanne impressed his friends and reporters by having them board 70 boats and then towing the boats through choppy water, swimming a distance of $1\frac{1}{2}$ miles, while handcuffed and shackled. Although exceptional, Jack's feat helped demonstrate the importance of keeping fit and active as we age.

3. Enjoy Your Sex Life

A discouraging mythology about sex among the aging would have these poor folks giving up sex for the most part in the later years. However, the Starr-Weiner Report, questioning over 800 people between the ages of 60 and 91, has revealed that 97 percent of this group enjoyed their sex lives and 75 percent considered their sex lives at least as or more enjoyable than when they were younger.

4. Keep Your Lifestyle Young

It appears that remaining fit as a fiddle into those special extra ten years has more to do with lifestyle than with any intrinsic physical limitations. Consider, for example, the careers of basketball great Kareem Abdul Jabbar, golfing legend Jack Nicklaus, boxing champion

George Foreman, Olympic swimmer Mark Spitz, and star pitcher Nolan Ryan. All five continued to perform superbly in their respective careers beyond age 40.

5. Slow Down as Little as Possible

Making these extra ten years as healthy and fit as possible begins by extending the fitness of our young adulthood as much as possible, and slowing down as little as possible over the passing years. Let's look at the example set by Nolan Ryan. In his mid-forties, Ryan struck out his 5500th batter and won his 314th game.

6. Maintain a Healthy Routine

Beginning in his twenties, Ryan maintained a successful, ongoing routine of healthy eating and exercise. After each game, Ryan worked out on his exercise bike. On days between games, he swam, sprinted, and did a goodly number of sit-ups. He makes it all sound so simple: "All you have to do is become more active and watch what you eat."

7. Never Allow Yourself to Become Inactive

The elegant simplicity of it is in the ongoing nature of such a lifestyle over the passing decades, even into the 60s, 70s, and 80s. One research project studied 184 healthy but inactive people over the age of 60. Part of this group began an exercise program while the remaining members of the group remained inactive. Of these inactive individuals, after the passage of two years, 13 percent exhibited new heart problems. Of the exercisers, only 2 percent showed such problems.

DAILY EXERCISE ROUTINES—THROUGHOUT LIFE. How better to have a sense of control over one's life than to be as physically fit as possible! Daily exercise routines that are enjoyable can be carried out throughout all of life, and are just as important to "successful aging" as they are to the earlier stages. At 65, 75, or even 85, we may have less vim and vigor, but still maintain a sufficient store of energy to continue to enjoy whatever physical exercise we choose.

Whenever I run my 5K or 10K Saturday morning races, I always keep an eye out for senior runners. If possible, I create an opportunity to chat with these inspiring individuals. In their 60s, 70s and 80s, these wonderful individuals continue to run competitively and, in the process, gain the benefits of "successful aging." Their sense of control over their own lives is much greater because of their enhanced physical strength and endurance. And this, in turn, can play a role in adding years to life, as well as adding life to years.

MEN'S LIFE EXPECTANCY IS GREATER NOW THAN EVER BEFORE

But how long can we remain competitive runners? The simple answer is *ten years longer.* A more thoughtful answer has to deal with the question: Ten years longer than what? Although my promise in this book is ten years longer than if you didn't follow the recommendations I propose, there is growing evidence that ten years of longer life may be a modest expectation.

Mean Lifetime Potential—110

Writing in the *Journal of Human Evolution*, Richard Cutler has calculated the mean lifetime potential (MLP) of various animal species, based on rate of development, length of reproductive period, and brain size. According to Cutler's calculations, the MLP of humans is 110 years.

"Life Endurance"—114

This surprisingly high figure is in rough agreement with that of Kenneth Manton of Duke University who analyzed extensive U. S. Census data to determine the "life endurance" of Americans.

Average Life Expectation by 2050—100

And finally, citing data from the Census Bureau, Paul Siegel and Cynthia Teauber report similar findings: "If the average annual rates of decrease in age-specific death rates recorded in the years since 1968 continue to prevail in the coming 65 years (to 2050), the average life expectation would approximate 100 in that year."

Life "Begins" at 65

Now you may more easily understand why the title of this chapter proclaims: "Growing old, staying young." Living ten years longer is no mere fantasy. Instead of living to our 60s, 70s, or 80s, we can in all reality look forward to even more years of "successful aging." Up to 100 years or more, according to the above-mentioned research.

Some of the accounts of the long-living individuals of the Soviet Caucasus are mind-boggling as well. Perhaps in a few cases, the truth has even been stretched by some individuals (as intimated by Alex Leaf in a *National Geographic* article). But the exact numbers relating to specific individuals are dwarfed by the number of large group studies and the actuarial projections of historical facts gleaned from national data banks.

For example, an individual claiming to be 138 years old was found to be lying about this significant feat. When the proper documentation was uncovered, it turned out this individual was a "mere" 101. Not bad!

But what really count are the studies that focus on large groups rather than accounts of individuals. In his book, *Who Shall Live?*, Victor Fuchs compares two adjacent states—Utah and Nevada—with similar climates and topography. He found that, despite the similarities, deaths from cirrhosis and lung cancer were two to six times higher in Nevada than in Utah. Were the Nevadans being punished by Providence for their evil, gambling ways? Not quite. Closer to reality was the realization that Utah is populated largely by Mormons, whose religion forbids smoking and alcohol. Across the United States, Mormons live 30 percent longer than their fellow Americans. So this statistic alone suggests that you can hope to live at least ten years longer just by following the suggestions from my chapter on smoking. Following the remaining suggestions on nutrition, fitness, and so on, should virtually *guarantee* the additional ten years I promise.

WANT TO LIVE LONGER? THE CHOICE IS YOURS!

The point here is that we *can* live substantially longer according to research on healthy lifestyle: we *tend* to live longer if we have a sense of control over our lives; we *will* live longer according to actuarial projections based on U. S. Census data.

"But," you may ask, "if the data project additional years in my life, why bother working at it myself? It'll happen regardless of what I do!"

Not quite, my friend. It'll happen to some and not others (more across the board, of course). If you want to be among the long-living, then you can choose to do so by improving your lifestyle along the guidelines suggested in this book.

It all adds up to this: As time goes by, as a group, we can anticipate living longer lifespans. This means that, although this is true for the group, those individuals who make certain lifestyle changes are more likely to be longer-living than the rest.

"LONGEVITY POTENTIAL" TEST

In order to determine where you presently are in the process of gaining ten more years of happy, healthy living, you can take the following test.

Each area of realizing your longevity potential is covered over the 20 items listed. There is a 5-point scale so that you can make the most accurate estimate of your own lifestyle. If for any reason you cannot answer a certain item, just circle the "3" in the middle of the scale. For example, if you have no idea what your cholesterol level is for Item 9, just circle "3." Then add up all the circled responses to get your total. The test will allow you to compare your score to those of your friends or others in your family.

After you've finished reading the book and have had a chance to start making changes, you can take this test again to see how much you've changed. Take the test every 3 months or so to see how you're doing. That way, you can monitor your progress over time.

"Longevity Potential" Test

1. Do you feel in charge of your life or a victim of circumstances?

in charge				victim
5	4	3	2	1

2. In general, do you feel stressed or relaxed?

relaxed				stressed
5	4	3	2	1

3. In general, do you feel confident or overwhelmed?

confident			overwhelmed	
5	4	3	2	1

4. In general, do you choose to eat high-fat foods (cakes, cookies, beef, sauces) or low-fat foods (pasta, vegetables, rice, fruit)?

low-fat				high-fat
5	4	3	2	1

5. Have your attempts at dieting ended up with weight gain instead of loss?

no				yes
5	4	3	2	1

6. Do you consistently take a vitamin supplement?

yes				no
5	4	3	2	1

7. Do you enjoy a healthy sex life?

yes		abstaining		no
5	4	3	2	1

8. Do you manage to exercise three or more times a week?

3 or more		once a week		never
5	4	3	2	1

9. Is your cholesterol level over 200?

140		200		240
5	4	3	2	1

10. How many cigarettes a day do you smoke?

0	10	20	30	40+
5	4	3	2	1

11. How many ounces of alcohol per day do you consume?

0-2	3	4-5	6	7+
5	4	3	2	1

12. Do you make use of sunscreen to avoid exposure to the sun?

always	usually	sometimes	rarely	never
5	4	3	2	1

13. Are your relationships supportive?

yes				no
5	4	3	2	1

14. Do you generally communicate well at a deeper level?	always				never
	5	4	3	2	1

15. Do you consider this stage in your life as good or better than any previous ones?	yes				no
	5	4	3	2	1

16. Do you usually get the medical check-ups suggested by doctors?	yes				no
	5	4	3	2	1

17. Do you usually see a doctor if you sense something may be wrong?	yes				no
	5	4	3	2	1

18. Do you find yourself worrying much of the time?	no				yes
	5	4	3	2	1

19. Do you enjoy being sensitive to others' needs or do you feel others should be more sensitive to your feelings?	sensitive to others			others sensitive to me	
	5	4	3	2	1

20. Do you feel you have a sense of purpose in life, or do you often feel lost and confused?	purpose			lost and confused	
	5	4	3	2	1

SCORING

Total your points: _____   Points

Likely to increase your lifespan by ten years.	90–100
Likely to increase your lifespan by five years.	80–89
Unlikely to change your lifespan.	70–79
Read this book carefully.	60–69
Make this book your constant companion.	50–59
Call your doctor immediately!	40–49
Have you completed your will?	20–39

CHRONOLOGICAL AGE VS. BIOLOGICAL AGE

"When I turned sixty," actor Paul Newman thought out loud, "I got into a real terrible funk." Then he flashed one of his famous smiles, "But I was delighted to learn it was only the flu." How does this life-long star feel about turning 70 just this past year? "I'm just getting going!" he shot back.

Jimmy Carter, another inspiring example of robust maturity, continues to excel in new ventures since leaving the presidency a decade and a half ago. Not only a very active international peace-maker in his years of retirement but, in addition, a successful published poet. In a poem entitled "Some Things I Love," from his book, "Always a Reckoning, and Other Poems," he mentions some of what still keeps him youthful:

> . . . The fight and color of a rainbow trout,
>
> . . .
>
> The end of a six-mile run in the rain,
> Blue slope, soft snow, fast run, no fall . . .

George Burns, in his late 90s at the time of this printing, knows full well how to discover when you're getting old: "When you resent the annual swimsuit issue of *Sports Illustrated* because there are fewer articles to read," or "When you find you're no longer worried about being involved in a paternity suit."

Scientific Proof That You Can Become 10 Years Younger

Although each case is different, two researchers, William Evans and Irwin Rosenberg, authors of "Biomarkers," have performed studies on 623 individuals who "tested biologically older than their chronological or calendar age—many by ten years or more." The evidence in these studies shows that within four months, the subjects were able to reduce their body age by over eight years. They looked younger, reached ideal weight, and reduced the number and depth of facial wrinkles. They felt better, and had more energy and enthusiasm for life. The conclusion of this research: "People in their fifties and sixties are as able to lower their body ages as people in their thirties and forties." More than 96 percent of the subjects ended up reducing their biological ages.

PROFILE OF A MAN WELL OVER 100

So how can you live a more healthy lifestyle to keep yourself youthful and happy as you grow older and stay younger? Well, let's look to those familiar folks in the old yogurt commercials. Scientists have studied the lifestyles of the long-lived individuals of the Checheno-Ingush Republic in the Northern Caucasus. Those living in the mountains had less than one tenth the number of strokes and about one-tenth the number of heart attacks as those living down in the plains. There was six times as much hypertension in the plains as in the mountains, and twice as much as in the foothills.

Those Who Live to 90: An Unhurried Pace of Life

Why were the mountain folk so much healthier? Those living in the mountains were much more likely to be in a "good mood" or positive mental disposition. These were individuals who lived to 90 or more. Eighty-three percent of these long-lived mountain men were pastoral and agricultural workers living "an unhurried pace of life."

One outstanding example was Medzhid Agaev, 133 years old at the time of study. A shepherd who was still following his herd 10 to 12 miles daily, Mr. Agaev had no mortgage or car payments to make, no business deadlines, and no traffic to fight (except for an occasional misdirected sheep). He, along with 91.4 percent of his mountain-dwelling compatriots, never changed their occupation. Nor had he or his compatriots changed their very moderate eating habits throughout their lives. Four times a day, Agaev would eat small portions of cheese, vegetables, yogurt, honey and fruit. He drank only spring water.

The Importance of Support Systems

Kinship and family network are, for Mr. Agaev and his friends, very important support systems that provide the basis for stress-free and meaningful lifestyles into old age. So marriage helps to provide the continuity of a supportive network of ongoing relationships. The worst possible curse in this culture: "Let there be no old folk in your house to give you wise counsel, and no young people to heed their advice."

Wanted: Elders and Younger Folk

It may not be essential in our culture to be married to enjoy a longer life, but a reliable group of friends, some elders you can count on for sage advice, and younger folk who respect and appreciate your opinions, certainly help.

According to Hans Selye, author of the classic book, "The Stress of Life," stress "accelerates the rate of aging through the wear and tear of daily living." Medzhid Agaev and his countrymen aged at a very slow pace. Part of the reason was the minimal amount of stress in their lives.

Stay Stressed, but Avoid *Distress*

Minimal stress does not mean inactivity and passivity. It means the absence of *distress*, as Selye uses the term. Stress, the enjoyable kind, can be healthy, as in sexual excitement, social excitement, or physical challenge. In that sense of the word, you *want* to stay stressed as you grow older. It's the distress you want to avoid—fear, anxiety, alienation, depression. One important way of keeping challenging stress from becoming distressing is to ensure the support of close friends around you.

THREE STRESSBUSTERS FOR LONGER LIVING

1. Counseling

At least having one person in whom you can confide the deepest, darkest secrets of your life is an essential starting point. If you don't have the time or excess energy to devote to finding such a relationship, you can still find support in our culture; the process is known, of course, as counseling or psychotherapy.

2. Social Group Involvement

It's important to feel accepted and appreciated by at least one social group, be it a church group, social group, or professional society.

3. To Lose Anxiety, Be Honest

Finally, it's important to be honest with yourself. "To thine own self be true," wrote Shakespeare, and you can be false to no other human. By being honest with yourself, and fostering a relationship of honesty and integrity with others, fear and anxiety become exceedingly rare companions.

With less fear and anxiety, there is less distress on the inner workings of the body, and therefore a healthier immune system and a very strong component in the realization of ten younger years of life.

SCIENTIFIC EVIDENCE THAT YOU CAN LIVE WELL OVER 90

So staying younger as you grow older involves being able to depend on others and having others depend on you, in a supportive network that reaches in both directions in terms of age.

That's what contributed in good part to longevity among the long-living residents of the Caucasus. In a group studied in the mountains of Daghestan, there were over ten times as many long-living individuals (past the age of 90) in the mountains of the Gumbetov region, where life is rural and stress-free as in the cities of the plains below. At the time of the study, there were 187 nonagenarians for every 10,000 individuals in the mountain areas and only 17 in the cities below—more than ten times the number of folks over the age of 90.

Stay Interested in Life as You Get Older

In this study, the nonagenarians in the mountains of the Northern Caucasus were far more active and more interested in life than their shorter-lived counterparts in the lower levels.

Sula Benet, who lived among this population for months at a time, met a 107-year-old man who said, "I am not old yet. I am in good health and working. I will be all right yet for a long time to come." After meeting scores of such long-living people, Benet concluded: "In the Caucasus, people feel that as long as they are in good health, working, and functioning in their social roles, they are not old."

Even fertility and child-rearing can go on into old age. At the age of 90, Gadzi Murtazaliev married for the third time and subsequently fathered 13 children. According to his wife, Zagidat, "He never cursed, even when exasperated. He considered a peaceful life, without quarrels, the greatest blessing."

SECRETS FOR LONG LIFE

Part of the secret of this stress-free society is the socially supportive aspect of sharing meals. According to author Benet, "Feasts are occasions for peacemaking with enemies, establishing friendships, and creating good will. Past differences are often resolved, new relationships are formed, and discordant elements are brought into harmony with the well-ordered structure of living so important to the Caucasian people." At such feasts, the eldest are given the seats of highest honor, while the young "stand around the table in readiness to serve the needs of the adults."

How different from our own North American culture, where the elderly are seen as unproductive, inflexible, and senile. According to the Pulitzer Prize-winning book, *Why Survive? Being Old in America*, by Dr. Robert Butler, old people (yet certainly younger than 90!) are considered uninteresting and condemned to a socially limited lifestyle. "There is . . . a greater debasement, a debasement based on loss of self-esteem, of significant social roles, and of a sense of importance."

Create the Conditions of Support in Your Own Life

I, myself, have considered moving to China when I reach my golden years. There, old age is revered, and respect grows with the passing years—just the opposite of North America. But a more practical approach for most of us would be to take a lesson from these cross-cultural comparisons. By building close and supportive networks into our social structures, we can take responsibility to create the conditions for our own increase of lifespan by ten youthful years.

A study of 7,000 California residents revealed that those with smaller social networks were two to three times more likely to die in a nine-year mortality follow-up than those with larger social networks. If we understand that larger social networks provide a more stress-free world for us to enjoy our lives, it is easy to see how such psychological factors can influence our physical health.

Beyond the foods we eat and don't eat, the supplements we take, the exercise we do and the support networks we nurture, it is mind-set and attitude toward life that help determine how long we live. How we see our reality, negatively or positively, is important. Focusing on the negative obviously makes our inner world more negative. Conversely, focusing on the positive makes our inner world more positive and, by extension, creates the groundwork for growing old while staying young. This cannot be achieved by having a pessimistic, depressed frame of mind.

What is critical for a strong attitude that allows us to stay young is the sense of control we feel we have in both our decisions and their consequences. If I feel in control of my life, then my stress level is much lower, independent of all the stress factors that impinge on my life.

Frustration can result when an individual begins to feel that he has no control over his life. If I see myself in charge of my life and in control, I feel strong, capable, and confident. If, on the other hand, I experience the events of my life as beyond my control, I feel more and more frustrated. A sense of helplessness that is learned early in life and persists over time can lead to a pessimistic attitude and, in addition, can be counterproductive to a long, healthy lifespan. So living ten years longer requires a take-charge attitude in which there is a feeling of control over most of life's challenges.

Why Meeting Challenges Leads to Confidence

What is crucial here is that you get a sense of controlling the specifics—the rewards—in your life precisely because of your determined efforts, not because of something over which you don't exercise personal control. For example, if you experience rewards for protracted effort, then you can acknowledge and take glory in the success of your efforts. On the other hand, if you experience rewards because of something other than your efforts—say, an inheritance or natural good looks—a multitude of rewards gives little satisfaction.

WHAT IT TAKES TO STAY YOUNGER WHILE GROWING OLDER

Staying young requires an optimistic, take-charge attitude that gives you a sense of control over your life and your physical health. It's quite ironic that the happiest periods of many men's lives occur when they are relatively poverty-stricken and struggling. When were you happiest? Probably at a stage in which you were struggling your way to success rather than at a time when you were enjoying the fruits of your labor. The reason is quite simple. You get the deepest satisfaction from life when the effort you extend brings about a reward that is highly meaningful. If you put out tremendous effort with little result, you can be frustrated and cynical. If you put out little effort but get tremendous rewards, you can be bored and cynical. But if you put out great effort and achieve tremendous results, you'll probably feel proud and successful. If there is a direct correlation between effort and results, you can feel meaningfully involved in life—otherwise, you may feel frustrated or bored.

If there is an absence of relationship between your efforts and the results—no matter how hard you try, you get nowhere fast—and if that happens often, especially in your youth, then you may acquire what psychologists call "learned helplessness." The more in charge and confident you feel, as you'll soon see, the healthier your immune system, and the longer you'll tend to live.

In order to avoid learned helplessness, it's important to know yourself well enough to take on challenges that you can master confidently, increasing the degree of challenge as you grow in your rate of success and confidence.

Master the Basics

What's most crucial, initially, is to master the very basic skills of the challenge you undertake, and then to move on to slightly more challenging steps very gradually. If you would like to play professional ball, then you must start with very basic throwing and catching, over and over. If you would like to be a comedic entertainer, then you must start telling a single joke over and over to different people until you get the nuances and timing just right before you move on to another joke and then another, and so on. The key is to break a skill down to its basics and then to do it until that initial step is mastered.

Spend the Most Time on the First Steps

Most of us don't have this discipline, despite the fact that it's a very simple one to describe and understand in theory. A friend of mine wanted to be a successful tennis competitor. No problem! He bought himself a machine that lobbed tennis balls out to him at various speeds and angles. Sure enough, after practicing for many, many hours on this patient, reliable machine, my friend was able to compete with the best.

Feeling in Charge Can Lead to a Longer Life

To explore the very specific relationship between confident optimism and function of the immune system, scientists at the University of Pennsylvania in 1987 studied 47 individuals between the ages of 60 and 90. They took blood samples from these people and examined the ratio of "helper" cells to "suppressor" cells, a high ratio indicating a healthy immune function. The results: The higher the degree of healthy optimism, the stronger the immune system.

As further proof that a confident, optimistic approach to life boosts the immune system, another scientist found that optimistic college students were less frequently ill than pessimistic students (3.7 days versus 8.6 days) and had to visit their doctors less frequently (once a year versus 3.6 times a year). Is it any wonder that Norman Cousins was able to cure himself of a debilitating collagen disease by watching funny movies from his hospital bed!

Acquiring *Self-Efficacy*

One way of looking at optimism as a result of achieving successful results through determined effort is what psychologists refer to as *self-efficacy*. This is defined as an individual's belief that a certain behavior will result in a particular outcome, clearly an indication of self-confidence. A man with self-efficacy is more likely to be successful in taking on the challenge of living a healthy lifestyle, and consequently be more likely to earn ten extra years.

So how do you begin to choose a path of self-efficacy that leads to a longer life? Just tap into your inner Fountain of Youth for ten more years of healthy life.

Step One: Choose a Supportive Environment

Choosing successful experiences in childhood would be an excellent start. But since we can't go back in time, where do we start now? We do so by choosing to be with people who are supportive and encouraging. It's been illustrated that students often react to teachers' expectations of success or failure. We often respond to others' subtly expressed expectations of us, even as adults. By choosing a supportive environment around us, we set the stage for self-improvement and a growing sense of confidence.

Step Two: Find a Buddy

For starters, look for a close, trusted partner with whom to share your new adventure. This individual will offer encouragement and realistic, honest feedback as you pioneer this new path. If both of you decide to begin together, all the better. You can be each other's support and feedback system all rolled into one good partner.

Step Three: Find Your Master

Another way to increase self-efficacy is to choose models or mentors who teach us by example or by instruction. We can choose to learn from those who already know. If that individual isn't available in person, we can watch from a distance (as in classes or lectures), obtain videotapes of him (or her) or read about him or her. Having a mentor is extremely helpful.

Step Four: Take Action

Once you've chosen an area on which to focus, whether it be a social skill, a healthier way of eating, an athletic or intellectual skill, or whatever you decide upon, take *action*. You may not be as comfortable as you'd like when starting a new behavior, but here are a few tips to help you along the way.

GIVE YOURSELF BIG REWARDS FOR SMALL STEPS AT FIRST. Start slowly. Take little steps at first. Give yourself (or one another) big rewards for small beginning steps. Think of an automobile engine. First gear moves slowly but takes a lot of fuel. By the time you get to fourth gear, and the car's already picked up momentum, it takes much less fuel to move quickly over greater distances. If overdrive is available, the car is speeding along with minimal fuel consumption. So give yourself (or one another) a lot of fuel in terms of reward and encouragement during the beginning phases. As time goes by and small successes lead to larger ones, you can ease up on the need for reward and encouragement and just allow time to share success stories and look for the new challenges.

BREAKING THE ICE——"FAKE IT 'TILL YOU MAKE IT." One of the challenges in beginning a new skill or habit is that it doesn't feel familiar. Of course not! If it did, you wouldn't be exploring new territory. At this point, many feel that since the new behavior doesn't feel familiar or comfortable, then it's experienced as phony—not the "true me." This is often used as an excuse to avoid trying this new experiment. "It's just not me," you might find yourself saying. "It's not in my personality."

Well, here's where the nuts and bolts of self-efficacy come in. It's your decision to choose something new—to improve your life—that can now prevail, to replace poor habits that lead to disappointment and a discouraging sense of helplessness. So if you have to "fake it until you make it," then do so. If you're so overweight that jogging makes you bounce all over and embarrasses you, then walk at first, in a mall or airport instead of at a track or spa. If crowds scare you and you decide to become more social, then attend low-key social gatherings at first, concentrating on one person at a time. Learn to do simple things such as acquiring a firm handshake while smiling and making eye contact, such as allowing yourself to be curious about this new person and allowing your questions of interest to flow naturally. Virtually all people enjoy talking about themselves to someone who has a genuine interest. Don't forget to give yourself (and each other) lots of credit for these simple yet challenging steps.

MASTER EACH STEP THOROUGHLY BEFORE MOVING ON. Stay with the first, early steps a bit longer than you'd like. Don't move ahead too quickly. Allow yourself sufficient success with the beginning steps till you become slightly bored with them. That means you've mastered them thoroughly; they're no longer the challenges they once were. Now you're ready to move ahead to the next level of challenge, whether that means walking/jogging on a track or telling a single joke to the new people you've met after you've chatted about yourselves. Enjoy your mastery of each beginning step before moving on. In acquiring self-efficacy, moving slowly is much more efficient than speeding ahead before you've mastered the step at hand.

Step Five: Keep Track of Your Progress

Keep aware of your progress in some systematic fashion. The best way to do this is to keep some sort of chart, using some measure of progress. It's amazing how rewarding it is to actually see your progress in chart form, so you can actually count (on) your successes. Success breeds upon itself, as does failure. So even if your successful steps are small (as they should be), it's important to be able to see these successes at a glance—the more frequently, the better.

Step Six: Learn from Your Mistakes

Another way to enhance self-efficacy is to manage your emotions. By that, I mean to understand your feelings and acknowledge this truth, both through introspection and by getting feedback from trusted friends. When frustrated and angry, acknowledge these feelings initially and then let them go. Replace them with a curiosity as to how events led to the frustration. What could you have done to avert failure? Once you discover the answer to that question, don't blame yourself but, instead, consider yourself the wiser and more able to glean success from similar circumstances in the future.

Step Seven: Stay Honest

The healthiest communication style for enhancing self-efficacy is assertive honesty. Holding back on the expression of one's needs is unhealthy and actually life-threatening. Life expectancy is strongly influenced by a resilient and resourceful psychological makeup. The more self-expressive we are, and the more self-efficacy we bring about in our lives, the longer we can expect to live.

Step Eight: Choose Your Own Lifestyle

Across the ages there have been periods when individuals have had more self-efficacy than others, and it is during these eras of "personal power" as opposed to collective subjugation that people added years to their lives. In the Middle Ages of Europe, for example, when the opportunities for individual expression and personal choice were at a minimum, life expectancy was low. On the other hand, as we currently experience a period of growing personal power and individual rights, the normal lifespan is growing in years. One of the components of this trend to longer life is the opportunity for individuals to choose their own lifestyles, and to explore different habits of eating and fitness.

Despite the large amounts of money spent by the food industry on advertising fast foods and snacks that are too fat, too sweet, and generally unhealthy, more and more individuals are choosing to decrease their consumption of such foods and the trend seems to be in the direction of a healthier eating lifestyle. Personal efficacy in this case means choosing healthier food despite a cultural influence in the opposite direction. The more in control of their lives people feel, the more they can express themselves, the more their rights are protected, and the longer they will live.

Step Nine: "Give Away" Your Success

Become a giver in your area of success. There's no better way to lock in success than to share it with others. If you've discovered something that contributes to your health, let others know about it. If you're becoming more physically fit, offer to assist someone else in his struggle. If you're gaining in social confidence, support those who are as shy as you once were. Just don't be fanatical about it. Offer, don't "push"!

Earn Success and Increase Your Confidence

Success breeds success. The important thing is to get started, obtain the proper encouragement and share your successes with others. The more control we have over our lives, and the more we become aware of such control, the healthier we become. Stress is reduced the more we feel in control, independent of the degree of actual sources of stress. To put it more simply, it's not the problems that determine your stress level. The more control you're able to exert over your life, the more confidence you gain, the healthier you become. Remember that riches or good looks in themselves don't lead to self-efficacy. It's the effort expended and the resulting success that makes you confident, happy, and healthy. Handsome models who rely solely on their looks and rich people who have inherited their wealth (and then choose to lay back and just spend all the money) can now be more easily understood as victims of circumstance. They just haven't had the experience of testing their abilities. So their confidence in their inner character (putting looks and money aside) cannot grow. As a result, these individuals may become quite dissatisfied with their own lives despite their outward trappings of material success.

Don't Just Read This Book, Live Every Page of It!

This book is broken down into chapters that cover varying components that contribute to living ten years longer and looking ten years younger. As you achieve success in one area, you're more likely to achieve success in another. It really doesn't matter where you start. As you gain success in including the right supplements in your vitamin and mineral intake, you'll feel more confidence about eating less fat. As you begin to achieve the level of fitness through exercise that feels right for you, you'll feel more devoted to avoiding cancer by eating more fruits and vegetables and staying on top of detection procedures. As all this makes you feel better about yourself, you begin to take more pride in your long-term appearance and manage to stay out of the sun or remember your sunscreen. You begin to support others in your social network by helping them make their lives longer and more youthful. You even consider contributing the benefits of your personal success to the public at large by writing for your neighborhood newspaper or our *Live Longer Newsletter.*

As it all comes together, you begin to realize, through your decisions, your actions, and support of others, that looking ten years younger and living ten years longer is really nothing more than taking charge, no matter how challenging the circumstances—gaining access to that inner Fountain of Youth.

Those lifestyle changes that are most likely to lengthen our lifespans and enhance the youthfulness and good health of those added years are clearly spelled out in this book. But simply reading the words on the pages provided is not going to do it for you. Here's what will:

TEN-POINT LIFESTYLE PROGRAM

1. Find a friend or family member with whom to share your lifestyle changes.

2. Share this book with your new partner.

3. Take the time to support one another.

4. Learn these four affirmations on which you can meditate:

   a. "My entire body feels ten years younger and I feel as sexy as ever."

   b. "My choices in lifestyle, grooming, and skin care allow me to look ten years younger."

   c. Choose an affirmation of your own that relates to your love life. Think about what you'd most like to have to feel better and focus on that. For example, "I choose to enjoy great sex with my partner by creating the right opportunities for that," or "Every day I choose to make a positive difference in my lover's life."

   d. Choose an affirmation of your own relating to a personal goal, such as losing a certain number of pounds, or increasing your speed on the jogging trail. This should be a goal that you can measure easily and that is fairly easily attainable. For example, "I can feel myself becoming thinner and expect to lose two pounds by next month," or "I can feel my body becoming more fit and expect to be able to keep up with my jogging partner by the end of the month."

5. Spend at least one-half hour a day relaxing with your lover and sharing your best self in an emotionally intimate way.

6. Make a personal commitment to three hours per week of your favorite exercise in any combination you like.

7. For the next six months, select one chapter from this book and make that chapter your companion for the month. Read it, reflect on it, and try its suggestions on for size. At the beginning of the next month, select any other chapter. Don't necessarily go in chronological order. Select the chapter that appeals to you most at the time.

8. Forge ahead on all fronts slowly but consistently.

9. Compare notes with your partner and support one another's progress. Focus on improvements in health and appearance. Celebrate your successes together: have a healthy meal at your favorite restaurant, enjoy great seats at the game, create a weekend away.

10. After six months or so, whenever you feel you've achieved substantial change, choose your own way of sharing your success with others: by volunteering to help others less fortunate than yourself, coaching at your local high school, teaching, or writing, perhaps. There's nothing better to "lock-in" your hard-earned successes than sharing them with others.

When all is shared and done, you too can look ten years younger and live ten years longer. All it takes is a decision, one that can change the entire course of your life and your health.

The great end of life is not knowledge, but action.

—Thomas Huxley

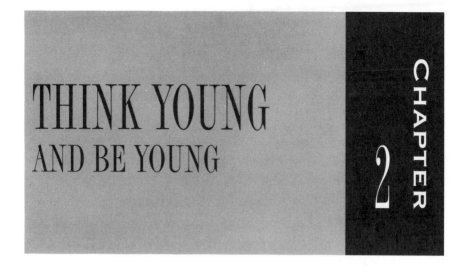

THINK YOUNG
AND BE YOUNG

At the age of 91, Dr. Benjamin Spock, happily married to a woman 40 years his junior, had this to say about his old age: "I don't feel great, but until two years ago I didn't even feel old."

AGING AND THE POWER OF THE MIND

Staying young and healthy has much more to do with what goes on in the mind than what happens at a physical level. When Dr. David Spiegel of Stanford University compared two groups of cancer patients—one with standard treatment and the other with standard treatment plus weekly support-group sessions—the support group not only suffered less pain, anxiety, and depression but also, quite surprisingly, lived *twice as long*. A review of the literature proves this to be consistent. Married cancer patients, for example, live longer than their unmarried counterparts.

Dr. Dean Ornish, as well, pioneered work with heart patients who were able to have their heart disease reversed (something the medical community had thought impossible until that time). They not only reduced their consumption of fat radically and took up physical exercise; they also formed a tight-knit support group amongst themselves wherein, with the full support of a caring doctor, they were able to unveil their deepest fears and self-doubts. They talked about their fear of death, their deepest misgivings and what their lives meant to them in the final analysis. When Dr. Ornish was asked what component of the program was most essential, he answered that none was. It was the whole enterprise of commitment to a new way of life, including not only nutrition, fitness, and support groups, but also yoga, meditation, and a new respect for life and loving relationships.

In my own cross-cultural research as I traveled through Europe, Asia, and the mideast over a three-year period, I found that the healing of illness took place when two belief systems coincided—that of the healer with that of the "patient." Across the various cultures, both contemporary and traditional, when a "patient" believes in the healing process he undergoes and the doctor/healer/monk is also convinced of the process, then the "patient's" health improves.

In the Middle East, I once sat on a dirt floor, sharing a meal with Arab nomad chiefs. I visited ancient churches in the Holy Land, and sought out the high priests to learn their esoteric secrets of the healing power of faith. Atop an old Arab structure, with the desert sun beating down on our heads, I debated intensely with a Hasidic rabbi about the relative benefits of ancient versus modern lifestyle and their effects on longevity.

In China, where I taught Western principles of psychology, I witnessed the healing powers of traditional herbs and acupuncture. In Hong Kong, at a Taoist temple on a misty mountain top, I was introduced to the mystical healing powers of the Tao. In a Thai temple, not far from Bangkok, I entranced Buddhist monks with the powers of hypnosis while they enchanted me with the magic of meditation.

The healing process seems to reside within the "patient" himself and just needs the permission of his society, as represented through the healer, to allow the healing process to do its "magic" work. After all, the body is in the process of self-regeneration all the time, as long as the individual is alive. Some ritual, characterized by prayer, a special potion or herb, meditating on the mystical Tao to the smell of incense, the rattling of bones or an expensive hospital stay, says to the individual's regenerative and immune processes: "OK, body, it's time for you to heal yourself. Everybody's looking at you and waiting. Drop everything else and get to work!"

This fact is well known in our modern age and by the contemporary medical community. It's referred to as the *placebo effect*. This can best be explained by the fact that when an experiment is done and one group gets the treatment and the other doesn't, even the non-treated group improves, precisely because the group *believes* it's getting the treatment.

My belief is that the same can be said for the aging process. If you believe in getting old quickly, your body processes will accommodate you. You'll feel older, you'll do the things expected of an older person, you'll give up on keeping your body young through proper nutrition and fitness, and you'll look older in terms of your demeanor and appearance.

Cure Cancer by Laughing It off

It turns out that one of the key factors that contribute to aging is stress, or how you deal with it. Grief and depression are often the precursors to such autoimmune diseases as rheumatoid arthritis. Even cancer is affected by the emotions. In his popular book, *Anatomy of an Illness*, Norman Cousins was able to cure himself of terminal cancer by exposing himself to as much humor as he could get hold of, whether in funny movies or humorous books.

Stress Pioneer Fights Off His Own Cancer

Even Dr. Hans Selye, the pioneer of stress research, was able to cure himself of a type of cancer by committing himself to "try to squeeze as much from life now as you can . . . because I'm a fighter, and cancer provided me with the biggest fight of my life." Although doctors gave him less than a year to live, he went on to live a full and productive life for another 10 years, dying a natural death at age 75. In the words of Dr. Bernie Siegel, author of the best-selling *Love, Medicine and Miracles*, "Exceptional patients refuse to be victims. They educate themselves and become specialists in their own care."

In one sense, this book is all about gearing your *mind* to the possibilities of living longer and looking younger, even more than it is about gearing your body in that direction. As your mind goes, so will your body. Each chapter of this book will engage your mind first, before you will engage your body.

According to the latest research, measures of mind function have been found to be even superior during the 50s and 60s than in younger years. Contrary to popular belief, the mind stays young, functioning even better through the 30s and 40s and through the 50s and 60s, before it begins to decline, at least in perceptual speed and numeric skill, in the 80s. Why not make use of this increasing youthful quality of the mind to enhance a more youthful body?

In Chapter Three you will learn how to use meditation and yoga to turn back the aging clock. There's no limit to how you can make use of these disciplines. The "hunger pangs of success" and the affirmations to help you become a nonsmoker, which you'll learn about later in the book, are slightly different forms of meditation, in the sense that you'll be using your mental powers to convert a destructive habit to a constructive one. You can also use yoga and meditation to reduce stress so that your arteries start shedding the layers of cholesterol that have accumulated over the years.

Afraid of doing something as "weird" as yoga and meditation? Well, if you think it's more acceptable to work so hard that your increasing stress level results in open-heart surgery, then that's certainly one choice that's available to you. Frankly, I think it makes more sense to spend some time each day on such enjoyable and simple exercises than it is to give someone the permission to cut open your rib cage to play "sew-the-pieces-together" with your one and only heart. "Thinking young" is much less expensive and not nearly as frightening.

Beyond that, would it surprise you to learn that there is no consistent evidence in the research literature that open-heart surgery prolongs life? That's right! Neither does angioplasty, where a balloon is inserted into the arteries to squeeze away the blockages. What such surgery does do is lessen the chest pains and discomfort that these individuals suffer, but three major randomized studies have proven that such surgery does *not* prolong life.

However, when you make a choice to change your lifestyle so that you take care of your body through proper nutrition, exercise, and a greater appreciation of relationships with other people, then you choose to take control of your life rather than sign it away to a hospital. And being in charge, feeling a sense of control over your life, is what enhances your health, strengthens your immune functions, and allows you to live out your potential lifespan, possibly into the 90s, but at least into the 80s.

EXTENDING YOUTH: APPETITE FOR ADVENTURE

Living ten years longer involves a commitment over time—continuing your "three-times-a-week" fitness routines, eating to stay slim and healthy, and quitting smoking. Without this commitment, there is an irreversible, inevitable change that occurs over time: A slowing down of energy, a loss of youthful agility, increasing susceptibility to illness, and a witnessing of the aging process reflected in the mirror. Beyond looking and feeling ten years younger than your chronological age, there is still something else to come to grips with. That ten-years-younger look and body provide you with the opportunity for an adventure of extended youth. The challenges of living ten years longer are undeniable. Beyond the midlife crisis, there might be a mature-stage crisis, making the physical, emotional, and economic factors of the midlife stage pale by comparison.

A Second Life to Live

Once you've made the commitment to live ten years longer, it's almost as if you have a second life to live in terms of opportunities for a second career, a renewal of a relationship, the beginning or resuming of an artistic or creative calling of some sort. This "better-half adventure" can be a whole new life change in terms of values, with less emphasis on physical attractiveness, a more honest approach to relationships, a greater appreciation of the spiritual as opposed to the material. Realizing the shortfall of your earlier years, you can now make up for lost time.

The Sexual Shift

Psychiatrist Carl Jung has described the *contrasexual transition* that occurs at midlife. Men allow themselves to become softer and more intuitive. Women allow themselves to become stronger, more assertive, and more self-directing. Their sexuality may be freed up after menopause, no longer concerned with pregnancy. Once the children have left home, father's bread-winning role and mother's nurturing role can be abandoned in favor of less restrictive values and lifestyles. Hopefully, the couple can stay in tune with one another despite the transformations.

How to Enjoy Your Extended Youth

There's no doubt that your adventure of extended youth demands a certain degree of self-acceptance. Self-image can change. Allow yourself to appreciate the more unique character showing in your face. Give up hard-driving physical endeavors and take a more moderate approach to physical activity. Self-esteem can come from self-generated goals and accomplishments as opposed to externally awarded grades and promotions. Being recognized for competitive achievement can be replaced by the loving glow from the pleasure of seeing grandchildren or young relatives come into this world.

The Contentment Factor

There's something very comfortable about the more relaxed approach to the "better-half adventure." We mellow out, as is often said. I call it the *contentment factor*—that commonly acknowledged loss of intensity as we ease into the comfort zone of life. There is some medical evidence to fortify this assumption; between the ages of 40 and 60, scientists have found, there is a loss of cells in a part of the brain known as the *locus coeruleus*, a part of the brain which registers anxiety. What a pleasant gift nature has bestowed on us to make the "better-half adventure" more enjoyable!

SIX YOUTH-EXTENDING ACTIVITIES

1. Call a Halt to the Madness

The first half of life one is on a constant treadmill. According to a Harris survey, leisure time has shrunk, since 1973, by 37 percent. During this same period, the average workweek has grown from 41 hours to 47 hours. The more ambitious professionals may end up putting in more than 80 hours per week, flitting from one stressful demand to another. Now, in the better half of your life, you can finally call a halt to such time-squeezing madness. You can relearn to enjoy life's leisurely pleasures—savoring the nuance of an old wine, enjoying the unrushed pleasure of a newborn grandchild, getting lost in a juicy, historical novel, or just plain ol' watching the sun actually set.

2. Enjoy the "Harvest Years"

The "better-half adventure" allows you the grace to return to the world what you gained in whatever good fortune you've had till now. Psychologists refer to this as the stage of generativity. You can now enjoy the continuous, ongoing process of life rather than a series of unrelated events. You can begin to connect with others because you care for them, not because you're forced to out of social or economic obligation. You can finally afford to live out the authentic values you have always talked about in the abstract. You can now afford the time it takes to reconnect with your inner self, just by taking the space to relax and meditate.

During these "harvest years," you can bring together all your experiences to discover and express your special uniqueness to those you love and about whom you care. You've reached the prime of your spiritual life.

Accepting the concreteness of your mortality, you can savor each day for its precious opportunities for love and joy. Secure in the appreciation of your own values, you can now allow those different from you to be themselves without your having to judge them. You become more tolerant of differences.

3. Find the Meaning in Your Life

In midlife, you question the meaningfulness of your career, the occasionally-felt emptiness of your life, and even the love in your marriage. Now you can reaffirm your close relationships, find your true calling as a vocation or hobby and create the meaningfulness in your life you deserve.

Your search is for completeness. If you devoted the first half of life to career, you now have the freedom to find the nurturance of intimacy. If you chose to be a devoted, nurturing father, you now have the freedom to unleash your drive to achieve a personal goal. If you wandered as an uncommitted, free spirit, you can now go back home or at least rebuild as much of it as you're able. Your quest is for wholeness, to bring back the missing part of your earlier half.

NAPOLEON DIDN'T GET IT. Too many commit the error of attempting to amass as much power over others as they can. A good case in point is the story of Josephine and Napoleon. He chose to build his Grand Army to conquer Europe and then attempted to overrun Russia as well, only to be beaten by the forces of nature as much as the fury of the defending Cossacks. "General Winter" and "General Famine" crushed his army with a more severe blow than could the Russian forces alone. But while away from home pursuing political gains, his wife, Josephine, grew further and further from him, so that when he finally did return home, he had to plead with her to be allowed into their bedroom. The conqueror of all Europe, head of the Grand Army, and yet a miserable beggar outside the door of his own bedroom. Ultimately, he was rejected by the presiding political forces, and exiled to the island of Elba. Such are the deserts of those seeking the power to dominate others while forsaking those close to home. I share this story not to prove my point, but merely to illustrate it. Who else had amassed so much outer power and had so little personal power when confronted by his own wife in his own home?

PERSONAL POWER BEGINS AT HOME. Personal power does begin at home, and extends outward, rather than the opposite. One of the most powerful of the Ten Commandments is to honor your parents, and by extension, your family. As you enter the "better-half adventure," you come home again in a spiritual sense. Whatever your early experience of family life, you can begin the process of forgiveness by posing the question: What is the source of your better qualities and your inner resources? The answer has to be your family of origin. Whatever faults you can blame on your family, it is also the source of your best and finest qualities.

4. Choose to Spend Time with Those You Admire

Once you've made peace with your family of origin, you're more capable of choosing and nurturing those relationships which truly nurture you back. Choose those people you not only find attractive, but also whom you respect or admire. For it is with such individuals that you will find a shared value system and thereby the opportunities for greater personal growth. Choose the priority of sharing time with these people. And if you live far apart, take to the fine old fashion of letter writing. Take the time to share what's in your heart. Such relationships, carefully nurtured, can grow over the years, enriching your lives in a mutual way.

5. Become Your Own Artist-In-Residence

Allow yourself the luxury of becoming your own artist-in-residence. If you're musically inclined, buy yourself an instrument you've always liked and learn how to play it. Create your own music, to express the rhythms and melodies of your inner soul. If visual art is your medium of choice, learn or relearn your favorite medium. At the very least, give yourself the opportunity to decorate your own living quarters with whatever appeals to the inner you.

Before the renowned psychologist Carl Rogers died, I was visiting him at home and noticed a series of color photographs mounted on a prominent wall. In his 80s at the time, Dr. Rogers was able to express his aesthetic sensibilities with beautiful photographs of his own making. He had no need to rely on photographs taken by others or on the advice of professional decorators. Here on the wall of his living room was a view into his own heart. He was feeding his own soul on a daily basis by decorating his home with his own artistic expressions.

6. Become an Author-in-Residence

If you enjoy the written word, then you need no special instruments or equipment except for pen and pad or, if you're technologically inclined, a word processor or PC. You can write a newsletter pertaining to a particular passion of your own. You can write your soul-mate friends, giving yourself license to explore your inner self. At the very least, you can write to that most important individual: your very own self. We call it a diary or journal keeping. If you have a flair for the dramatic, try writing short stories about issues that pull at your heart strings. Or write a play—enjoy the fantasy that a producer will get hold of it, and beg you to allow him or her to make a film of it.

WRITE YOUR OWN STORY. I believe that everyone's life is worth a story. Explore your own issues, what makes you tick, what moral lessons are to be gleaned from your own life story. What really matters to you and what is to be done about it? If your life story points to some purpose, then this is the time for it to find expression, not tomorrow. Write your autobiography as if it were destined to be a best-seller.

Such self-expression and self-exploration can enhance the probability of living the full ten years longer and then some. According to Dr. Deepak Chopra, renowned author of *Ageless Body, Timeless Mind*, six traits in particular are key for longevity:

1. Responding creatively to change.
2. Reducing anxiety.
3. Focusing on the ability to create and invent.
4. Maintaining high levels of adaptability and flexibility.
5. Integrating new things and ideas into your life.
6. Wanting to stay alive.

Finding a creative expression of your unique self affords you the opportunity to create and invent, integrate new ideas into your life and respond creatively to change, especially if your creative outlet is in writing.

In order to manifest your desire to stay alive, become more adaptable and flexible, and reduce anxiety, it's important to reduce stress in your life. This leads to our next section on staying younger by reducing stress within your family.

HOW LOVE TURNS BACK THE CLOCK

Study after study reveals that having a close, supportive network reduces stress and promotes cardiovascular health. It's not only outside pressures that cause our blood pressure to rise; it's also the absence of supportive friends and family. Your closest relationships seem to matter most for your health. The more hostile you are during a marital argument, the harder it is on your immune system.

A study of stress using macaque monkeys produced similar findings. In it, the friendliest monkeys were found to have stronger immune responses while the more hostile and aggressive had the poorest. According to one of the researchers, "Affiliation protects animals from the potentially pathogenic influence of chronic stress."

Have at Least One Friend from Whom You Hold Back Nothing

The number of supportive relationships is not as important as the quality of those relationships that do exist. In a nutshell, the lesson here seems to be: Nurture at least one or two highly supportive relationships in which you can totally be yourself, divulging your deepest secrets, holding back nothing. That's better than having fifty friends, none with whom you can be completely open. And learn to be friendly, rather than hostile, cynical and mistrustful.

Learn How to "Fight Fair"

When couples fight for dominance, blood pressure rises. But when productive fighting occurs—in other words, to solve a problem rather than to gain dominance—blood pressure does not rise. "Fair fighting" skills can help you avoid destroying your health. Struggles for dominance can lead to heart disease, but if your relationships are a source of comfort, they can exert a protective effect on your heart.

DEVELOPING AN AGELESS OUTLOOK

You've heard that life begins at 40. In this book, you'll learn how life can last ten years longer with a healthier lifestyle. You've also heard how youth is wasted on the young. Whether or not this is true, this section is about not wasting the mature years of your life—that part of your life that starts today—and developing an ageless outlook.

As we mature, intellectually and emotionally, we learn to be less selfish, less centered on our own needs. Having spent our youth on a narrower perspective of humanity, we're now learning that a much deeper joy can be acquired by taking on a wider perspective of life. As we mature, it feels much better to be able to give of ourselves to others, supporting others emotionally, spiritually, and intellectually. We can be more prepared to take time to be aware of others' problems, to let them know that we care and to impart the wisdom of our experience.

This change in perspective as we mature out of the more formative years of our lives not only nourishes others, it nurtures our own inner selves in very significant ways. As we learn to reduce stress in our lives through better communication with others, to be clear about our needs and to be sensitive to those of our loved ones, we enhance our physical health as well. By reducing stress in our lives we enhance our physical as well as mental health. As we acquire a more generous disposition toward those around us, we can look forward to a more meaningful and enjoyable longer life.

SENSE OF PURPOSE

One of the key attributes of happy, long-living men is a sense of purpose in their lives. No matter what else transpires around them, these men do not lose their own sense of direction.

A sense of purpose can be described in both general and specific terms. At the general level, most men would agree on a common goal—to have our existence make a difference, to make use of the talents within us to make this earth a better place because of our being here—and to find deep meaning in that endeavor.

On a specific level, how that mission is carried out differs with each individual, and may change over time within each person. For many years, I felt my mission was to help others deal with their life challenges through the art and science of therapy. Now it appears my mission is being manifested through the written word. I write not only books such as this, but dramatic pieces as well—both as a novelist and playwright. At this time of writing, only two of my plays have been presented; but by the time your read these words—who knows?

As part of my education for writing drama, I recently took a course on writing screenplays. One evening, the instructor made a fascinating point about dramatic structure which, as I thought about it, also applied to real life. The protagonist or hero of any drama typically goes through a transformation to a "higher" level of being, and this transformation is not made by conscious decision. Rather, it is made (usually in the third act of a movie) when, just as the hero seems to be overcoming the challenge at hand, the worst of all possible outcomes happens. The rug is pulled out from under his or her feet, the world is turned upside down, making the previous challenge look like an anthill compared to the newly challenging Mt. Everest. Now the hero is ready for a *real* transformation.

If you recall the film, *Kramer vs. Kramer*, Dustin Hoffman's character loses his wife because he is too focused on his job. His challenge is to learn to release his tight grip on the career ladder and to learn to have a loving relationship with his son, who is now his sole responsibility. Much of the film has to do with this early transformation from corporate climber to a truly caring and loving father. Just as he completes this painful transformation, what should occur but the most terrible possible outcome. His wife reappears and decides she wants her son back!

The Greatest Lesson—Discovering What We're All About

Think about your own life. Would you agree that only when the worst possible outcome challenges you, are you really forced to change? It is at such times that we are more open to discovering our inner purposes in life. The greater the challenges in life, the greater the lessons to be learned in finding out what we're really all about. It's the universe's way of getting our attention with a two-by-four upside the head, demanding: "Is this what your life is really all about? Wake up and look around!" We don't always make major changes through conscious decision. Life forces us out of our ruts and demands that we look around for a more meaningful path.

With Age, We Find More Learning Opportunities

As we get older, more learning opportunities are created for us, through failed relationships, professional setbacks, medical problems, and so on. Yet each cloud has its special silver lining—even the thunderstorm clouds. As we mature, we're forced to explore our purpose.

Joy Comes from Day-to-Day Relationships

As we mature emotionally, we may begin to realize that joy comes not from things, such as fast cars and wall-sized TV screens, but rather from the humble process of day-to-day relationships and how we choose to use our productive time. It's no longer the end result that matters as much, such as plaques on the wall or getting the better of someone, but rather the ongoing process of enjoying the relationships we do have and enjoying our work and play on a daily basis. Shakespeare says it so eloquently:

Things won are done, joy's soul lies in the doing.
—Troilus and Cressida, Act 1, Scene 2

The More You Offer, the Less You're Hurt

The more open you are to exploring your deeper purpose in life, the less you will need "most undesirable outcomes" to get your attention. The more you can embrace a sense of purpose, the less you will be susceptible to "most undesirable outcomes." The most selfish individuals are those who are trying to hold on to control of their own lives and those of others—they are most susceptible to life's challenges. Those with a sense of purpose, generally to make available to others what they can offer, emotionally, spiritually, and intellectually, are least hurt by life's challenges. We can call this *Ryback's First Inverse Law of Giving*: The more you have to offer life, the less you're likely to be hurt by life. The same events may happen to the giver and the taker—illness, emotional loss, financial setback—but the giver is less hurt by such events.

Givers Tend to Be Healthier, Less Greedy, and Well-Liked

The giver's eyes are set on the purpose. As long as giving is still possible, whatever its medium, then life is still rich and meaningful, and illness, material loss, or personal insult take on a relatively minor role. Paradoxically, however, those with a deep purpose of giving, in some form, to others are more likely to remain healthy, free of material attachment, and well-liked by others. As we live a healthier, vital life for ten or more years, it makes more sense to learn the deeper purpose of being a giver rather than a self-centered taker.

Give to Others—You'll Feel Less Alone

Other than physical harm, the greatest source of stress is the sense of alienation we experience in life. A sense of purpose of giving to others removes that sense of alienation. As we give to others, whether it be through teaching, listening, or just being there for those who need us, we feel a connection with the life source and we become less susceptible to loneliness and rejection. We become less needy of material acquisitions and external symbols of achievement and more appreciative of the love and honesty we develop in our relationships and the comfortable sense of leisure that comes from enjoying whatever happens to be around us. We can enjoy our love for others, in its various forms and manifestations, as well as the challenge to discover what special qualities or talents are unique to us as we choose to use them for the betterment of others, no matter how small that betterment may be. And, as Demosthenes pointed out:

> "No man can tell what the future may bring forth, and small opportunities are often the beginning of great enterprises."
>
> **—Ad Leptinem**

Enjoying the Inner Self

The more we can rise above our petty desires and lift ourselves to the greater common good, the more we can trust our inner feelings to be true guides of our own behavior. Some call this intuition, others call it gut reaction. The more we free ourselves of petty desire and vulgar competition, the more sensitive we become to that inner guide that, over time, proves itself more accurate than intellect and logic. We become more comfortable with ourselves and enjoy time alone as a special treat rather than as loneliness. We may even choose to spend time with our "inner" selves, in gardening, music, or meditation. Paradoxically, people seem to be more drawn to us now that we need them less. *Ryback's Second Inverse Law of Solitude*: The more you learn to enjoy your solitude, the more people are drawn to you.

Giving Is Continual Fulfillment

There is so much we can attach ourselves to in terms of material objects or goals of achievement. We can never be satisfied if we continue to look away from ourselves, from our own inner resources. External desire knows no end. A "house" as a symbol of success and achievement is never completed—it always needs more, to impress our neighbors. A "home" is accepted as it is—for its warmth and character, not to impress others. So it is with our lives. To impress others, we will never be completely satisfied. To have as our purpose to give to those around us, our lives are continually fulfilled. Harriet Sewall writes of this so beautifully, in her poem, *Why Thus Longing*:

> "Why thus longing, thus forever sighing
> For the far-off, unattain'd, and dim,
> While the beautiful all round thee lying
> Offers up its low, perpetual hymn?"

You Can Be the Source of What Others Need

To live in need is to live in conflict—conflict between your desires and those of others—as if the world were running out of what you need. To live with purpose is to live as if you are the source of what others need. By choosing to live with purpose, you do indeed offer what others need. As you choose to live a longer, healthier life, you have the supreme gift of enjoying a "better-half adventure" and helping those around you to enjoy their lives as well.

How to Achieve It

How can you achieve this sense of purpose? The answer is extremely simple. Just stake claim to it! Take this very moment and make a claim to aspire to the purpose of offering yourself first to your loved ones—your mate, your children, your parents—and start becoming aware of others' need for your love and acceptance. It's not your money or your cherished possessions or your time we're talking about, though they probably want at least some of those items.

Don't Stop Yourself from Showing Love

At a deeper level, they simply want to be accepted and appreciated by you. You probably do love and appreciate them, but are you preventing yourself from showing it? So the first step is to start with those closest to you.

Second, make peace with yourself. Learn to be more honest with yourself. Give up comparing yourself to others. Accept your shortcomings and allow yourself to become more appreciative of your uniqueness. There is no one exactly like you, never was, never will be, and this makes you uniquely special. Treat yourself to the experiences you really want, the music you like, the honesty you deserve with those you care about, the relationships with people you admire. Get to know your quieter self by spending quality time alone, in artistic pursuit, walking in nature, or just meditating in whatever way you most enjoy. By treating yourself as someone special, you'll begin to accept no less from others. You'll have less time for those who don't make you feel special. The quality of your life will grow in quantum leaps.

LIVING MORE FULLY

Your fears will begin to dissipate, leaving you only with the inevitable fear of death and taxes. If you don't cheat on your taxes, that leaves you only with the fear of death. Here's *Ryback's Third Inverse Law of Living Fully*: The more fully you live your life, the less will you fear your death.

The more you put off for tomorrow, the greater your fear of losing tomorrow. The more life you enjoy today, the less you fear loss of the future. By living on purpose, you make each day, each moment, more real and significant. Tomorrow is more opportunity to give more to others. Your death becomes more their loss than your own.

Empower Those Around You

As your mind-set shifts from neediness to giving, your present life takes on more meaning and the future is an opportunity for more of your giving nature. In addition, you feel that your inner energies empower those around you. What you give away to others will live on beyond your physical demise. Although that sounds very philosophical, you can begin to get a sense of it and you can begin to feel a timelessness about your life.

So the "better-half adventure" of your life is directly ahead of you. It doesn't necessarily begin at 40; it can begin today, regardless of your age. One thing's for sure, there's no more time to be wasted. To the extent that you can learn to be more of a giver for those extra ten years, you'll have all the more to look forward to. Remember: The more you have to offer life, the less you're likely to be hurt; the more you enjoy your solitude, the more others want to be with you; the more fully you live, the less you have to fear. So enjoy yourself. The better half is yet to come!

KEEPING YOUR MEMORY SHARP: FOUR QUICK TIPS

Enjoying your "better-half adventure" not only keeps your heart younger and healthier, it also keeps your mind active and healthy. The ability to remember, reason, and solve problems is superior in those over 60 who continue to exercise their faculties to the fullest.

As you age, neurologists say, part of your brain having to do with thinking and memory shrivels away at a rate of 10 percent per decade. Over a lifetime, the rate of transmission along neurons slows by about 10–20 percent. Yet, for those who stay fit, brain function can actually improve through middle age. How is this possible?

There are two reasons for this. The first is that the brain is full of redundant circuitry. There are many times the number of neurons we need to function at top level. So even though there is loss of brain process, there's more than enough left to pick up the slack.

The second reason is that the brain can be made to grow new neural connections through intellectual stimulation. Mental exercises can actually make the brain grow new nerve endings and more than make up for the losses due to aging. "Use it or lose it" describes the situation well. Challenge your brain and you'll stay steps ahead of any loss due to aging. Here are four tips that will assure you a top-functioning brain.

1. Expect to Communicate Even Better as You Mature

According to neurosurgeon Vernon Mark, recently retired from Harvard Medical School, the mature person's brain can be prone to decline in certain complex areas of intelligence such as theoretical mathematics. However, intelligence in areas of applied skills does not decline, and certain areas such as art interpretation increase with time. Speech and writing abilities can actually improve through the 50s and 60s. Philosophers often don't hit their stride until age 70 or 80.

2. Add Mental Workouts to Your Physical Workouts

In addition to physical exercise, mental exercise also helps keep the brain in tip-top shape. To complement physical exercise for the body, consider the following mental workouts for top brain functioning.

Occasionally, balance your checkbook without the aid of a calculator. This will improve concentration and attention. If your mind is not otherwise occupied (during phone conversations, unimportant meetings), practice the fine art of creative doodling. Working playfully at geometric designs or simple cartoon-like drawings will improve perception of spatial relationships as well as enhance creativity. You might even graduate to the point of taking up drawing or painting, a wonderful creative expression that can be enjoyed into your 70s, 80s, and 90s.

3. A One-Minute Memory Course

Memory can become problematic as you mature. One way of compensating for such loss is to combine a component of memory which does not decrease—music and verse—with the logical memory which does tend to decrease with age. By putting the items you would like to remember in lyrics of songs you know very well, you can improve your memory beyond its original, younger state. Another technique, advocated by many memory experts, is to assign the numbers 1 through 7 to the various parts of your body (for example, 1 = head, 2 = eyes, 3 = mouth, 4 = chest, and so on), and then associate items you wish to remember with those numbers and body parts. Silly associations are not only allowable, they're encouraged. If you have a grocery shopping list to remember, just imagine each item growing out of the assigned part of your body, and let yourself be silly about it. Imagine a loaf of bread growing out of the top of your head, pears for eyes (a pair of pears), pearl onions for pearl white teeth, broccoli growing on your chest . . . . . I'll leave the cucumber to your imagination.

4. Roy G. Biv—the Use of Acronyms

Another memory technique is the use of acronyms, taking the first letter of each item to produce a nonsense word which is easier to remember than the list. You don't have to wait until you start losing your memory to age to begin acquiring this skill. A superior memory is desirable at any age. I can still remember the colors of the rainbow from the acronym "Roy G. Biv" I learned in elementary school—red, orange, yellow, green, blue, indigo, violet. Without Roy's help, I could never remember the definite order of the colors. From college, I remember the acronym OOTAFAGVSH for the spinal nerves without hesitation, though the individual nerves don't come back as readily. Optic, trigeminal, facial, glossopharyngeal, vagus are all I can remember, not having thought of this for many, many years. Yet how amazing that I can recall that much after so many years in an instant, with the help of an acronym! The more you practice this, the more you'll have access to this lifelong skill. And so your memory will be just as good as ever, for the rest of your life.

FOUR LIFE-EXTENDING QUALITIES

Such grace in the "better-half adventure," whether in making love or completing a personal project, does not fall gently upon us, but rather is a natural consequence of personal choice and determination. Left to our indolent and mindless habits of laziness, we can certainly expect the worst of aging with all its infirmity of body and vapidity of mind. But to take action against the evil ravages of old age is a powerful choice for extended youthfulness. Old age can certainly be a bitter and debilitating experience. Until our current generation, that's how it was considered typically. Certainly it has been thought of in this manner for centuries. Here's how Cicero considered it hundreds of years ago:

> As I give thought to the matter, I find four causes for the apparent misery of old age; first, it withdraws us from active accomplishments; second, it renders the body less powerful; third, it deprives us of almost all forms of enjoyment; fourth, it stands not far from death.

Meeting the Challenge of the "Better-Half Adventure"

Rather than a depressing dictum of dire decline, I see Cicero's comments as a challenge. If, during those special ten years, we can, first, stay active; second, remain powerful both in terms of body and mind; third, enjoy such powerful activity; and fourth, stay vital and engrossed in life rather than contemplate the inevitability of death, then the "misery" of "old age" can be transformed into the sweet experience of enjoying the "better-half adventure," freer than ever to explore our talents to their fullest, to share our love without reservation with family and friends, to push the edges of our vitality in whatever directions we choose.

Stay Vital, Loving, and Engrossed in Challenge

Early in his career, the comedian Steve Martin once confronted his audience as it sat laughing uproariously at his zany humor: "Why are you all so happy? Don't you know you're all going to die someday?"

This sobering question only provoked more laughter, as well it should. Death is just as inevitable to the helpless infant as it is to the person of years. There's no advantage to hastening its approach nor to considering our demise too eagerly. By staying physically active, socially involved, and enjoying such activity to the fullest, no matter what our age, we defy Cicero's "apparent misery." We stay vital, happy, engrossed in the challenges and successes of life, maintaining our own health and energy through active choices, loving those closest to us openly and honestly and supporting our friends and colleagues with the full use of the experience and wisdom of our years.

In celebrating his 75th birthday, General Douglas MacArthur shared with his audience the following description of youth, attributed to Samuel Ullman of Birmingham, Alabama:

> Youth is not a time of life—it is a state of mind. . . . It is a temper of the will; a quality of the imagination; a vigor of the emotions; it is a freshness of the deep springs of life. Youth means a temperamental predominance of courage over timidity, of the appetite for adventure over a life of ease. . . .

> Whether seventy or sixteen, there is in every being's heart a love of wonder; the sweet amazement at the stars and starlike things and thoughts; the undaunted challenge of events, the unfailing childlike appetite for what comes next, and the joy in the game of life.

> So play well the game of life. Play it in your quest for fitness.

Celebrate the food you eat with creative preparations. Respect the rules that govern the health of your body. Treat your playmates in life with similar respect. Love to the fullest, each day of your life!

The next chapter, for a change of pace, will get you prepared to take the best advantage of the useful information and suggestions on how to keep yourself relaxed and free of stress in order to enhance your chances of living ten years longer. You'll learn how to assume a winning attitude of taking charge of the stresses in your life, and how to master the skills of yoga and meditation, to maintain a healthy lifestyle that enables you to look ten years younger *and* live ten years longer.

— CHART I —
CHALLENGES TO FEELING YOUNGER

Challenge:	Solution:
Feeling overwhelmed?	Smell the roses.
Feeling lonely?	With others, be yourself completely.
Does your life feel meaningless?	Discover the missing half of your life and allow it back in.
Is your life feeling wasted?	Choose to share what's important to you with those you respect and admire.
Feeling uncreative?	Decorate your own environment and play from your inner soul.
Feeling unrecognized?	Write the story of your life—for yourself!

— CHART II —
REMEMBER?
IF NOT, THEN LOOK HERE:

To Improve Your Memory of:	Try this:
What is communicated to you	Keep expressing yourself creatively
Important numbers	Group them two or three at a time
Artistic concepts	Doodle creatively

A long sequence of events

A long list of items

A long list of names

Put it to verse or music

Use parts of your body as imaginary storage points

Practice using acronyms

ANTIAGING
STRESS REDUCERS

The greatest enemy to living ten years longer is not overeating, or lack of exercise—although those play quite significant roles—nor is it smoking or alcoholism. No, the greatest threat to long life is *stress*.

Stress, associated with excessive feelings of competition, dramatically raises blood cholesterol levels and causes blood to clot at a dangerously accelerated rate. Men who are subject to this kind of intense stress are *seven* times more likely to suffer from coronary heart disease than their less stressed counterparts. Such stress-driven men, even if they are otherwise physically fit, are 2 to 3 times more prone to heart attacks than their relaxed counterparts.

Ongoing, intense stress of a competitive nature changes a man's internal chemistry. Even healthy men undergoing such stress are not able to rid their blood of fat absorbed from their food as well as their relaxed counterparts can. This abnormal accumulation of fat in the blood tends to cause red blood cells to clump together—a dangerous predecessor to heart attack. In addition, such stressed men produce higher levels of norepinephrine, the "struggle" hormone, which also plays a major role in coronary heart disease.

In other words, without any change in diet or exercise, men subjected to ongoing, competitive stress will suffer from higher cholesterol levels, higher blood pressure, and a greater susceptibility to heart attacks.

One of the body's responses to stress is to divert blood away from the inner organs (stomach, liver) toward the brain and muscles (the better to fight). As the liver continues to be deprived of blood, it can no longer do its job of removing and converting the cholesterol and fat from the incoming food. Instead, such substances remain in the blood and are soon deposited in the arteries, leading to cardiovascular disease. Living ten years longer is not only about eating smart and staying fit. It's also about how you think and feel.

The kind of stress I'm discussing here is part and parcel of the attempt to do more, achieve more, accomplish more in less and less available time while feeling that you're struggling "against the wind" in order to do so. If this sounds like you, then you're also likely to feel angry and aggressive much of the time, and feeling rushed almost all your waking hours.

You also hate to comparison shop, wait in line for anything, or be forced to slow down in traffic. You find yourself planning your next day's tasks while conversing with others because they talk so slowly. And if you're on the phone, chances are you're also fiddling with paperwork—signing checks or something similar. If you can identify with these characteristics, then this chapter is written especially for *you*.

Since you're typically feeling so rushed and pushed for time, let me offer you the gist of this chapter's advice:

1. Slow down!

2. Let love come into your life.

3. Change your mindset and make the time to read the rest of this chapter. You need it more than anyone else!

But the rest of us need it too. We men are all more or less subject to a number of myths that entrap us into stress-laden lifestyles, taking on more responsibilities than we have the time and energy for. If we don't tackle these myths head on, we subject ourselves to increasing stress over the years, eventually robbing us of those ten more years. Here's a list of some.

TEN LIFE-SHORTENING PERSONALITY TYPES

1. Mr. *Independence* accepts the belief that he should accomplish everything that needs to be done without any help from others. He sees help from others as an indication of personal failure. His myth: he has better control over his life if he avoids depending on anyone else for help.

Mr. Independence is full of tension, keeping his emotional cards close to his vest. In both social and work settings, he'll tend to be the self-designated problem solver. He's what you'd call an independent thinker, so don't try to change his mind—you'd be wasting your time.

2. Mr. *Pleaser's* delusion is that it's his responsibility alone to make everyone around him happy, denying his own needs. He focuses intently on what others expect of him and is eager to jump through their hoops, asking only, "How High?" If the demands increase beyond his capacity to meet them, he puts more pressure on himself and suffers increasing stress.

Mr. Pleaser is all smiles, covering up his inner tension. He's eager to undertake all that's asked of him, totally blind to the fact that his inner physiology is being damaged the more he impresses others with his "good-guy" image.

3. Mr. *Success* suffers from a lack of inner self-esteem and compensates for that by achieving and accomplishing all he can in the shortest time possible. He only feels good about himself when he can count the palpable rewards society gives him for his efforts. In a vicious cycle of hard work, ignoring his need for personal love and the encouragement by society for this pattern of behavior, he works harder and harder, becoming more recognized for his accomplishments, and finally self-destructs in one form (physical illness) or another (stepping on others' toes, unethical behaviors) at an early age. His myth: Work yourself to death. (And he does!)

4. Mr. *Mad*, true to his namesake, is always hostile and angry. He has the inner capacity to be lovable (as we all do), but he's never

learned to trust that kind of personal interaction. His personal belief is that people will either use him or reject him if he lets his guard down.

You can see the anger in the corners of his mouth and in his eyes. The closest he can come to a smile is a sneer. If you don't agree with him, watch out for his "pit-bull" reaction. His myth: Love can't be trusted. So keep up your guard. Will Mr. Mad live long? Not very.

5. Mr. *Helper* is a nice guy, but gives up so much of himself at the office that his personal life pales by comparison. He's always available to his clients. The more his pager beeps at home, the more important he feels. His myth: My value is how much my clients demand my time and energy. My family and personal life mustn't interfere.

At home, Mr. Helper acts more like Mr. Poop-out. He's all give at work and all take at home. His personal life is as exciting as yesterday's warmed-over breakfast. Behind his eyes is a bland nothingness—no real joy for life, only for work.

Meet a few more personalities, results of myths that also shorten their lives:

6. Mr. *Muscle* buys into the belief that he's strong enough to take on all physical challenges, from building his own home to digging his own garden. He sweats away from dawn to dusk and then continues to buy into his myth by lifting weights as his hobby. No challenge is too great for him as he works himself into an early death. Men are physically invincible.

7. Mr. *Stable* has answers for all the emotional concerns of those around him. No problem is too complex for him to handle. But deep inside, the pressures mount, for he takes others' problems very seriously. This self-imposed pressure grows slowly but cumulatively, until the pressure on his heart takes its unfortunate toll.

8. Mr. *Romantic* is always ready for sex, at least that's what he'd like his woman to think. So ready or not, here he comes (pun intended), enduring all the performance anxiety that goes with being at his

woman's beck and call. His myth: It's a man's duty to satisfy his woman *all the time*. Well, this guy's all heart, but his heart may need some vascular surgery before too long.

9. Mr. *Provider* takes good care of his family, even if it means holding down two part-time jobs in addition to his regular full-time job, while insisting that his able-bodied wife stay home and relax. Every year he goes deeper into debt making sure his children have the best that's available in clothing, automobiles, and so on. He himself has no need for money since he's always working, except when he's at home mowing the yard, or repairing that leak in the ceiling. His myth: A man must provide the best for his family at any cost. Unfortunately, the most expensive cost, ultimately, may be medical expenses for cardiovascular surgery.

10. And, finally, we have Mr. *Star*, the center of attention wherever he is. His stories are always the funniest, the longest, and have him as the central character, always winning out in the end. He never comes into a room; he always makes an entrance. If the camera's in his hands, it's always pointed at himself, sporting the latest fashions and his "Hollywood" tan. His myth: A man is only as good as he appears. Truth is, he looks great on the outside, and feels completely stressed on the inside. This man needs a strong dose of reality. Without it, he'll die young, still looking perfect.

Surely, you can see a little bit of yourself in at least some of these mythical personality types. I can see myself, at least a little, in practically every one of them. At different times, I'm *independent*, a *helper* in my profession, *mad* at being disturbed when I'm into my work, trying to *please* my editors, *physically* pushing myself to stay fit and lean despite the passing years, taking pride in my emotional *stability*, and being *romantic* when it's called for. I enjoy my *success* for which I strive, I hope I'm a good *provider* and if this book doesn't make me a *star*, I'll be disappointed.

So I sure could use some stress reducers to keep my blood pressure and cholesterol count down. You too? Well, let's see what we can come up with to reduce those aging stresses.

SIX SIMPLE RELAXATION ESCAPE TECHNIQUES FOR STAYING YOUNG

In addition to resolving conflict with your mate, getting close to your kids, and nurturing special supportive relationships, it's also essential that you develop some techniques to help you relax on your own. Here are some helpful ways.

1. Escape into Music

Choose a selection of music that's special to you for whatever personal reason, no matter if the music you choose is corny or off-beat—the more off-beat the better. Then make a time for about 15 to 30 minutes when you won't be disturbed and turn on the music as loud as you like. Sit in your favorite chair and just let yourself be inundated by the music, locking out the outside world.

Sometimes I choose old folk music from the '60s or '70s. Other times I choose medieval music that I never hear anywhere else. It's my world for those 15 to 30 minutes. I don't have to please anyone else.

2. Escape into Fantasy

Taking the same 15 to 30 minutes of undistracted isolation, get comfortable and close your eyes. (You may want soft music in the background.) Let your mind wander into your most delectable fantasy and enjoy your own private adventure. Just set up a scenario and then let your imagination take off on its own.

3. Escape into TV

Space out with your TV remote. If you're so stressed out you can't relax, then sit in front of the TV and flick through the channels until you find a program that's on your level of intensity and let yourself escape into it.

4. Escape into Self-Indulgence

Schedule a day or half-day in which you do exactly what you want to do (without breaking the law or hurting anyone, of course). Go to an afternoon B movie. Sit on a park bench and watch the birds. Treat yourself to a fine meal at an elegant restaurant. No one to please but yourself—at least for now.

5. Escape into Whining

Write a letter to an old friend or relative, pouring out your heart and stresses. Then decide to mail it or not—at least you got it off your chest.

6. Escape into Worry

If you're stressed by compulsive worrying, set aside a half-hour the same time each day to focus on your worries. If you're inclined to worry any other time, just relegate your worries to your designated "worry time" and get back to focusing on what you're doing.

SLEEP WELL AND AGE WELL

Although most of us need about 6 to 8 hours of sleep a night, a number of very high-energy people can get by on as little as 4. Scientists believe that a natural 24-hour cycle lets our bodies "know" when to go to sleep.

But to keep from being stressed out, we do need our nightly sleep. So if you have trouble falling asleep, here are some tips on sleeping well.

1. Keep a Regular Time for Going to Bed

Our bodies are really creatures of habit. If you go to bed at different times, your body may ask: "What the heck's going on up there? Will you make up your mind so we can get some regular sleep?" When you do go to sleep at a regular time, not only will you fall asleep more readily, but the sleep you get will be more restful.

2. Set Up a Routine As You Prepare for Bed

A bedtime ritual is very helpful to prepare both the body and the mind for giving up the day's activities. Look at it as a form of seduction, inviting both body and mind away from external stimulation to quiet aloneness. That's what prayers do for children, and some adults. Children may want stories read to them, adults will read stories themselves. Others do different things. The last thing Barbara Walters does before retiring is to write her list of things to do for the next day. I myself watch Nightline on TV and then read a magazine for a while before turning off the light. Create your own routine and stick to it.

3. Do Some Form of Exercise Each Day

I've noticed that whenever I have trouble falling asleep, its quite likely I haven't done my exercise for a day or two. If you do an active exercise (running or swimming) every other day, then at least do some stretching or yoga exercises (which I'll get into soon) on alternate days.

But don't exercise just before going to bed. That'll stimulate your body. If you must do something physical before going to bed, you can either have sex or, if you're not lucky that evening, take a nice, leisurely stroll.

4. Avoid Caffeine after 4 P.M.

Different individuals have different sensitivities to caffeine. If you're having trouble sleeping, become aware of your caffeine intake. Be aware that caffeine sometimes comes in surprising forms—not only tea but also chocolate, soft drinks, and cocoa. Here's a brief list of caffeine sources:

Coffee (1 cup, brewed)	92 mg.
(1 cup, instant)	65 mg.
Tea (1 cup)	50 mg.
Soft drinks (6 oz.)	20 mg.
Chocolate (1 oz.)	10 mg.

Instead, drink a glass of milk, which contains the relaxing amino acid, tryptophan.

5. Don't Depend on Alcohol or Pills

Alcohol may put you to sleep, only to cause you to wake a few short hours later, unable to fall back to sleep.

Sleeping pills will work at first, but then you adapt to them and you're worse off than before. You become dependent on the pills even though they start losing their effectiveness. You can't fall asleep with them and it's even more difficult to sleep without them.

6. Stay Cool Rather than Warm

Most people sleep much more soundly in cool temperatures. As long as your body is kept comfortably warm by sufficient blankets, you can sleep in very cold temperatures, and more soundly as well.

7. If You Can't Fall Asleep, Just Keep Your Eyes Shut

The few times that I've been so energized that I just couldn't fall asleep, I experimented by keeping my eyes closed, even though my mind wouldn't shut off. I decided to try resting my body, despite my awake mind. Try that for yourself. If your mind refuses to shut off, that's one thing, but why should your body suffer as well! Let your body rest in bed and ignore your active mind. Your body, and mind, will feel more rested the next day. And you'll probably get more actual sleep that way. You may not have control over your mind, but you certainly have at least that much control over your body.

8. Meditate Twice a Day

Sometimes you're just too tired to fall asleep. You're dead tired but your mind won't let go. You go to bed and you just lie there awake, your mind and body too tired to do anything, but unable to sleep. The solution here is to try the discipline of meditation. This discipline is not a cure-all for everything, as some claim, but it's a lot better than whatever comes second. What meditation can do is allow you a couple of rest periods during the day so that you won't be so dog tired at the end of the day. Studies have shown that insomniacs can reduce the time needed to fall asleep from 75 minutes ordinarily to about 15 minutes after having practiced meditation for 30 days. In the next section I'll explain exactly how to learn the practice of meditation and how the benefits can help you reduce aging stressors.

HOW MEDITATION TURNS BACK THE CLOCK

Meditation has a deep, rich heritage, dating back thousands of years into Indian history. The "wisdom of the Himalayas" was brought to our familiar shores by the 89-year-old Guru Dev in April of 1959. Soon after, a very devoted American, Jerry Jarvis, poured his energies into bringing meditation to the attention of Americans. Jerry and his wife, Debby, gave talks to nearly-empty rooms until the interest in meditation began to grow very rapidly. Some time in the mid-'70s, the number of meditation practitioners reached the million mark, aided by the fact that the Beatles became devotees.

There are a number of ways in which meditation can help turn back the aging clock—primarily, though, by reducing stress in your life. Here's how meditation counteracts stress:

1. Relaxes the blood vessels, lowering blood pressure and eliminating a cold, numb feeling in the extremities.

2. Slows down the heart.

3. Slows down the breathing rate, with shallower breaths, reducing oxygen intake significantly.

4. Decreases sweating (a sign of tension).

5. Decreases the level of lactate (the result of fatigue) in the blood by at least 30 percent.

Here's a brief summary of the scientific findings on meditation:

1. When compared with sleep, meditation was at least twice as effective in lowering oxygen consumption; this was accomplished within minutes of meditation, while it took hours of sleep to do so.

2. During meditation, the number of breaths per minute went from 14 to 6.

3. As measured by galvanic skin response (a scientific measure of sweating), individuals became extremely relaxed during 20 minutes of meditating.

4. The pulse rate of meditators was less than 70, even when not meditating, as compared to a pulse rate of just below 80 for nonmeditators.

5. After at least 4 weeks of practice, the blood pressure of hypertensive meditators went from 150/92 to 140/85.

Even stressful anxiety was reduced while self-sustaining confidence was enhanced:

6. On two psychological tests of anxiety, meditators became less anxious by factors of 23 percent and 17 percent, respectively, within $6^1/_2$ weeks of starting, and by factors of 34 percent and 36 percent, respectively, after 43 months of meditating.

7. On another psychological test, these same meditators, after $6^1/_2$ weeks of meditating, became less depressed by a factor of 38 percent, less neurotic by a factor of 43 percent, and felt more self-esteem by a factor of 23 percent. After 43 months, these same individuals became even less depressed by a factor of 69 percent, less neurotic by a factor of 71 percent, and reported feeling more self-esteem by a factor of 67 percent. In another study, tests of memory indicated that, after 1 year of meditation, memory improved by 19 percent, and by another 8 percent after a second year.

8. When a group of prisoners was taught to meditate, a strong correlation was found between the total number of sessions and the degree of relaxation, according to David Ballou's report, "The Transcendental Meditation Program at Stillwater Prison."

9. For those prisoners who meditated regularly, their degree of psychological pathology (mental disorder) was reduced by 19 percent while they became more socially outgoing by a factor of 12 percent.

Proof Positive That Meditation Works

In a study specifically designed to see if meditation prolongs life in older individuals, 73 residents of retirement homes, with an average age of 81, were randomly assigned to one of three groups—one that practiced meditation, one that simply relaxed, and one control group. At the end of 3 years, over one third of the control group had died; $12\frac{1}{2}$ percent of the relaxation group had died; yet every single member of the meditation group was still going strong.

Ten Steps to Learning to Meditate

Meditation is a skill that can be learned fairly easily if you take the time and the space to do it and you're serious about your intent. All you need is a quiet space with a comfortable chair or pillow on which to sit, and 10 to 20 minutes of undisturbed solitude. Two options, although not essential, are highly recommended: some not-too-sweet incense and a pleasant-sounding bell or gong to mark the beginning and end of your sessions.

1. First of all, set the mood by appreciating the fact that meditation has been proven to slow down the cardiovascular processes and therefore can turn back the clock of aging within your own body.

2. Get comfortable in a sitting position you choose: either in a comfortable chair with your back and head comfortably straight with your head unsupported, or on a pillow with your legs in a lotus position with your hands resting on your knees. Take a few moments to get comfortable as you settle in. When you're ready, strike the gong to mark the ritual of the beginning of your meditation.

3. According to strict tradition, you need a special, personal "mantra," a Sanskrit word or sound used as a device to focus inward and block out the external world. Well, since our purpose is to turn back the clock of aging, I am going to assign to you a special device which will help put you in the proper frame of mind. I invite you to count backward very slowly—one count per breath—from 9 down to 1, then repeating the cycle. The "9" represents the decade of the 90s and each number down from

that represents the corresponding decade ("8" represents the age 80 to 89, "7" represents the age 70 to 79, and so on). This way, you can actually feel your age "slowing down," as your breathing and heart rate actually do slow down.

4. The first time or two you try this, you may find yourself engaging in what I call "mind chatter." Even with your eyes closed and comfortably seated, your mind may refuse to slow down and even challenges your attempt at meditation with cynical comments and questions of doubt. "This is ridiculous. I hope no one sees me. Why am I wasting my time with this silliness? What should I have for lunch today?" This is a normal process of the conscious mind's adjustment and will tend to disappear within a few sessions. Just ignore it and let it be. As you will with any intruding thoughts from then on, acknowledge the presence of such thoughts and then bid them a pleasant "good-bye" and continue to meditate on the decreasing numbers.

5. Although the purpose of your meditation is to turn back the clock of aging, other than counting backward from 9, don't focus on the goal. Instead, focus on the counting only and let yourself be drawn into whatever inner experience comes up for you. The more you can let go of conscious thinking, the deeper the process of meditation. Let the counting do it. All you need to do is nothing. And say a pleasant "good-bye" to whatever thoughts manage to break through.

6. You may find yourself drifting in and out of a state of semi-consciousness. Just let it be. Your conscious mind is always brought back to the counting backward. Say your pleasant "good-bye" to everything else.

7. Ultimately, you'll begin to experience more and more moments of inner, peaceful quiet. Enjoy those moments. At such moments you can feel a more youthful quality throughout your senses.

8. Let this youthful sensation sink deeper and deeper into your awareness. At moments, you can feel the clock of aging going backwards, making you feel younger and younger, but don't dwell on this feeling for more than a moment. Say a pleasant "good-bye," even to this, and return to your counting.

9. As you get more comfortable, you'll notice that your breathing becomes even slower. It's as if you're in slow motion. Your lungs fill quite slowly, filling up, up and up until they're completely full. Then, after a brief hesitation, they begin to let go as you exhale slowly and comfortably. As you breathe out, imagine yourself sinking lower and lower into your comfortable position, as if you were settling into the most comfortable bed. The lower you sink, the younger you feel.

10. Finally, as all this begins to happen more comfortably and more deeply, let go of all your expectations, concerns, and awareness and just let yourself be part of the in-and-out-ness of your breathing. Everything else will take care of itself. Each meditation may have a little surprise waiting for you. I don't know what it will be and neither do you. Just be open to it.

If you follow these guidelines, you'll become more skilled at getting into a deep, comfortable state fairly quickly. This meditation will not only relax you and fight the stresses that would otherwise contribute to your aging process, it will also condition your unconscious to be more receptive to the possibilities of living ten years longer and looking ten years younger. In addition to conditioning your mind in this direction, you can also condition your body as well. This is done with the help of the practice of yoga.

YOGA BRINGS RENEWED YOUTH

Your 30s are an excellent time to begin familiarizing yourself with yoga in order to maintain your youthful flexibility throughout your life, but whatever your age, begin now and just keep on enjoying it as the years go by. Let's begin with a few very simple yoga postures. These take very little time and can be done virtually anywhere, anytime, with absolutely no equipment, except for a comfortable spot on the floor.

Simply put, yoga involves the practice of assuming certain postures with your body. You will be using such postures to make yourself more flexible and limber for a renewed youthfulness. The key thing is to remember to build into these positions very gradually. Never strain yourself beyond what's comfortable.

For starters, all you need is a comfortable space on the floor with a towel or mat on which to lie if there's no carpet. Your clothing should be loose enough for you to do the postures without restriction of any kind. As for time, you can do it any time—morning, afternoon or evening—except for a period of about one or two hours after a heavy meal. I'd like you to commit yourself to doing the following postures on a daily basis for at least two months before you evaluate the results.

You may get stiff or your muscles may tighten up but don't give up—work through the discomfort. If all goes well, you'll not only feel more limber and more youthful; you'll also feel much healthier and more relaxed.

Incidentally, if you think that yoga's not manly, then think again. Hollywood hunks such as Harrison Ford and Richard Gere are strong devotees of yoga. You may not have their glamour, but at least you have a shot at their youthful vigor.

1. Knee to Head

Lying with your back flat on the floor (or a thin mattress or towel), bring one leg up, curling your knee and putting your hands over your calf, pull gently toward your body. Pull your head up gently to reach for your knee. Alternate with your other leg and repeat a few times. Be very gentle, especially at first. This simple exercise strengthens your stomach muscles, stretches your "hamstring" muscles and also strengthens the cervical, lumbar, and sacral parts of your spine.

2. The Frog

Here's another simple yoga posture. Sit on the floor with your soles together and your knees spread comfortably apart. Grab hold of your ankles and pull down gently, aiming your head down toward your legs. This simple exercise promotes flexibility in the pelvic area and stretches your inner thighs. These yoga exercises can be used to cool down after your aerobics.

3. The Cobra

Lie down on your stomach, legs and feet together. Place your palms underneath your shoulders, fingertips no farther than the tops of your shoulders.

Looking up toward the ceiling, raise your chest off the floor using your back muscles rather than your arms. Still using your back muscles, arch your back even more, feeling your belly button pressed into the floor. Relax into this pose and remain for 10 to 20 seconds. You can just feel your lower back pains disappearing.

Now, very slowly, return to the floor, turning your face to one side, and turn your hands over, palms upward, and relax for 20 seconds before repeating the entire pose once again.

4. The Locust

On your stomach with your arms out to the side, palms down, legs together, raise your chest up, eyes to the ceiling as you also raise your arms and legs off the floor. With your arms slightly backward, you may feel like an airplane trying to take off or like Superman in flight. Enjoy the sensation of "flying" for 10 seconds as you balance on the center of your abdomen, breathing normally. Make sure to keep your knees and legs together. At first, you'll find it easier to get your chest higher than your legs. That's okay. With practice, your legs will gain height too.

Come down slowly, turn your head to one side, turn your palms up and relax for 20 seconds. Then repeat one more time. The first few times you attempt this, stay up for only 5 seconds and build toward the 10-second interval. Like the cobra, the locust is also good for lower back pain.

5. The Half-Moon

Standing with your feet together, raise your arms over your head, palms together, thumbs crossed and locked. Keep your head up and your chin forward. With your arms tight against your ears, stretch for the sky.

Now slowly bend your arms and body backward as much as you can *comfortably*, keeping your arms straight, and breathing normally. Focus your attention on the back of your neck and relax into the bend.

Only after you've done this successfully for a few weeks should you attempt to continue to bend back even more. This is accomplished by pushing your thighs, stomach, and hips forward as much as possible.

At this point, you'll feel a stretching sensation in the small of your back. Breathe normally in this position, relax into it for a few seconds and then return slowly to center position. As you return, reach upward once again before beginning the next phase.

Now bend forward at the waist and grabbing hold of your lower calves, bring your forehead toward your knees. Eventually, you'll aim to touch your forehead to your knees but give yourself the time you may need to accomplish this.

Hold this pose for a count of 5 seconds at first and when you're ready, go to 10. As in all these poses, move as slowly as you like but do just a bit more each day.

Return slowly to center, upright position and lower your arms slowly and gracefully. After a few weeks of doing this once, repeat a second time. This pose not only rejuvenates many of your muscles but also improves the flexibility of the spine. It's quite like oiling the machine of your body, giving you an ageless feeling. The more you do it on a daily basis, the younger you'll feel.

6. The Soaring Eagle

In this pose, I want you to concentrate on breathing naturally and allowing yourself to ease into the pose, despite its challenge, so that you feel as if you were nestling into it.

Begin by bringing your right foot 4 feet to the right, raising both arms to your side, parallel to the floor, your palms facing downward. Point your toes forward and keep your knees straight but unlocked. The first few times you do this, you might want to have your feet five feet apart, making it easier for you, and then bring your feet back to the 4-foot distance as you feel more comfortable with the pose.

Now bend forward at the waist and grab the backs of your ankles firmly near the heel, all fingers together and thumbs on the outside of the feet, and bring your head lower and toward your legs. You'll feel the stretch in your hamstrings first. Now, instead of pulling with your arms, allow your upper body to fall naturally of its own weight and you'll be pleased to notice your head going even lower. Now is the time to relax and let yourself "nestle" into this position for 5 to 10 seconds.

Eventually, you can improve on this pose by making sure that your feet are only four rather than five feet apart, that your behind is pushed up further and that your head is hanging lower to the ground. Eventually, you want your head actually to touch the floor, but that may take a while. Once accomplished, you can enjoy relaxing into the tripod your body has created and just feel your youth being renewed.

7. The Relaxer

This last pose is your dessert. It's the easiest and most relaxing, yet just as important as the others. All you need to do is lie on your back, arms comfortably at your side, palms upward, with your legs comfortably apart. Close your eyes and let go of all the tension you possibly can, just imagining your body as heavy as possible. Imagine yourself a heavy piece of lead being fully supported by the floor. Enjoy for a few minutes or as long as you like, listening to soothing music if you like. This is one you can customize to your own likes.

If you can apply yourself to practicing these poses on a daily basis for at least two months, you'll begin to feel a definite sense of renewed youth. Your body will feel freer of tension, much more limber and healthier in general. You'll feel more balanced, not only in a physical sense, but in a spiritual sense as well. You'll have greatly improved the probability of your living ten years longer and looking ten years younger.

HOW TO QUIT WORRYING

1. Discipline Yourself to Worry Only at Specified Times

The opposite of meditation is worry. Just as meditation is good for you, worry is bad. So if you must worry, why not do so in a disciplined way! Instead of worrying at random, in an uncontrolled way, why not discipline yourself to worry at special worry times. You can take one half-hour a day, let's say at 5:30 P.M., and do all your worrying at that time. Any other time a worry pops up, you just say to yourself: "I'll just have to worry about that at 5:30," and then put it out of your mind until then. Of course, this takes discipline, like any other skill. Or you might want to reserve one-half day a week to deal with all your worries. For that half-day (I do mine on Friday mornings), you take all your worries and do what you can to solve them, then and there. Call people who can have a direct bearing on the solution of each of your problems, whether because of their expertise or special contacts. Don't gripe to those who can't be of any help. Make the calls to those who can help effectively, even if it's putting you in touch with someone else who can ultimately be of help. If you discover that no one can help you, then you at least know that that's so, and you can begin to look at other options.

2. Attack Your Worries Logically

Problem solving involves:

    a. identifying the problem clearly

    b. brainstorming all the possible options

    c. evaluating the best options

    d. aiming for the optimal outcome

The best problem solvers seem to find opportunities in the direst of circumstances.

3. Take a Pro-Active Approach

The most successful people tend to plan ahead and take a proactive approach to life rather than one that is reactive. Once you decide what makes you happy, you can form a goal—one that is specific, that you can accomplish, and that is exciting. Having specified a goal, you can now do the opposite of worrying, you can *visualize* your successes and, by doing so, begin to live out the small details that accumulate to the achievement of your goal—whether it's financial, emotional, or living longer in a more healthy fashion. By taking greater control over one of these areas, you assure yourself of ultimate success.

4. Visualize Success

By visualizing the successful achievement of your goals, you're creating the opportunity to mentally rehearse the steps necessary for success. Some writers refer to this as programming the unconscious.
Others refer to it as creative visualization, and still others as psycho-
cybernetics. Whatever you call it, it's been proven to work. Now,
experiment with your own goals and prove it to yourself.

HAVING FRIENDS HELPS YOU LIVE LONGER. In chapter eight on the
cardiovascular system, we'll be discussing the benefits of a supportive social network on longevity following heart attacks. But let me
mention now that in a study of 194 heart attack victims, those who
had two or more sources of emotional support were found to be
twice as likely to survive longer than a year after the attack than those
with no support.

A survey of six studies including over 22,000 individuals showed
that those with few friends or family had a death rate 2 to 4 times
greater than those of the same age with a rich personal network.
Reducing stress in your life by nurturing quality social relationships
helps you to live ten years longer. Just knowing they are there can
help. Merely feeling you have a safety net reduces your level of anxiety and gives you a sense of security.

I want to spend the rest of this chapter focusing on the family,
home, and career aspects of fine-tuning the stress factors in your life.

First, there is the need for reducing stress and conflict in your
close personal relationships. If you're a family man with children,
then the next section will address that as well. To reduce stress in
your personal life, consider making my suggestions an acquired
habit.

REDUCING STRESS AT HOME

The closest and most logical place to begin nurturing life-enhancing
relationships is at home, with your own family. If you're the father of
schoolchildren, the responsibility is yours to nurture open lines of
communication with them. Set aside at least one opportunity for

open discussion where you can catch up on their lives, so that they can get a sense of your place in their lives. The best, most logical time would be the evening meal. Not only is it essential for you to be on good, understanding terms with them; it's important for them as well.

How to Get Respect from Your Children

Another opportunity to strengthen the nurturing quality of family relationships is to have a family meeting to get consensus on all decisions affecting the family as a whole, whether it's getting a new pet or considering a move to another part of town. Letting the kids in on the process of decision making makes them feel important and makes it more likely they'll respect you as parents.

How to Achieve Family Closeness

Another way of enhancing family closeness is to develop some strong family rituals to help family members bond with one another. Don't overlook opportunities for family sharing such as holidays and birthdays. Beyond these conventional rituals, develop some that are unique to your family, such as attending Friday night football games if your child is on the team or in the band. Here's another, somewhat unconventional, way to stay in touch with your children in a special, ritualistic way: Get digital pagers for each member of your family and, as the mood strikes each of you, page one another with coded messages—111 for "I love you," 222 for "See you at dinner," 333 for "My allowance is due tonight," and so on. That's one way of using high tech to nurture close family ties.

ELIMINATING THE STRESS OF CONFLICT: SEVEN QUICK TIPS

The research on fighting with your mate indicates that too much or too little fighting is bad for your health. Here's why. Too little fighting may mean that at least one of you is suppressing your feelings, leaving you frustrated with suppressed anger. This can lead to high blood pressure and, over time, cardiovascular problems. Too much fighting means yelling, screaming, even physical violence, where more problems are created than solved. The key to better health and longer life is open discussion, possibly heated at times, that expresses feelings honestly, but also solves the underlying problems. Anger, when uncontrolled or unexpressed, is bad. Here's how to deal with your anger in a healthy, productive manner:

1. When arguing begins to become too intense or hurtful for either party, learn how to use the "T" sign for "time out" to take a brief breather.

2. Before arguing, get in touch with your own feelings, so you know what you want to express and what outcome you're hoping for.

3. When you do express your opinion, do so by taking responsibility, both for your actions and for your desires, rather than blame your partner. Instead of "Look at this mess you got us into," try "I did X which resulted in Y. Can you help me fix it, please?"

4. Make sure you've heard what your partner has said by paraphrasing what you heard to his/her satisfaction. "If I heard you right, you think that. . . ."

5. When you want your partner to change some behavior, clearly explain its effect on you: "When you do X, it makes me feel Y. Instead, would you consider Z?"

6. Don't wait for tensions to build so high that emotions take over, leaving no room for reason. It's much easier and less frustrating to plan on regular "pow-wows" to explore any differences of opinion that begin to come to awareness. Perhaps you can schedule one a week at a regular time, like Friday evenings or Sunday mornings. Then you can clear the air about whatever bothers you before you develop resentment and anger.

7. Above all, aim at common courtesy. Treat one another with respect. That'll go a long way in minimizing flare-ups.

Why "Good Fighting" Skills Are As Important As Sexual Skills

These rules are essential in virtually all relationships because of the complexity of man-woman communication. Male and female roles are not as rigid as they were a mere generation or two ago and so there's bound to be more confusion about responsibility and decision making. Both may want to have the final word on decorating the house even though their choices of style are 180 degrees apart. Both may have busy, successful careers, putting into question the division of labor around the house.

The family structure may be complicated if this is not a first marriage for either or both. Disciplining step-children can be extremely frustrating. Who has the final word on certain decisions affecting the children? Step-mother? Father? Biological mother? This is very fertile ground for family argument. Open communication and good fighting skills are just as important as good lovemaking skills.

STRESS-REDUCERS AT HOME: SIX QUICK TIPS

Stress can rear its ugly head at home, even in the absence of conflict. Here are some ways to reduce stress with very little effort on your part.

1. Unplug your phone when you need that alone time. Allow yourself a nice, long bath or an uninterrupted nap.

2. Instead of trying to remember all your household and yard work chores, write them down on a calendar so when the time comes you'll see exactly what's to be done and you won't feel stressed about forgetting anything.

3. Keep the top of your desk clean or at least organized. If you begin with a messy desktop, you'll never feel complete about any aspect of your work. So organize that mess at least once a month. Any task you then focus on will seem less stressful.

4. When giving or receiving directions, always repeat them to ensure their accuracy. A single wrong turn or missed street sign can cost upwards of a half hour. When giving directions, I always say: "Please repeat that back to me to make sure I didn't make any mistake." That way, I'm checking on myself, not the other person.

5. Clear up any stressful confusion by talking it out with a close, trusted friend.

6. Strive to be honest in your dealings with others. There's nothing so stressful as having to cover a lie, or worse yet, being caught at it. For less stress in your life, honesty is the best policy.

COMBATING STRESS AT WORK: TEN QUICK TIPS

1. Allow 15 extra minutes to make appointments.

2. Always have a magazine or paperback to read while you're waiting.

3. Don't schedule appointments back to back. Be realistic and allow for transition time.

4. Don't allow yourself to be over-dependent on approval for everything you do. Rewards are gifts, not the main fare. Seeking praise on a constant basis sets you up for frustration and stress.

5. Don't agonize over negative job performance appraisals. Learn from them. That's what they're for, not to create stress.

6. Give up the notion of maintaining total control. Don't try to meet every deadline and fill every quota.

7. Learn how to say "no" to extra projects that are clearly not essential.

8. Learn to delegate responsibility to capable others.

9. Allow for mistakes and judgment errors. Mistakes sometimes turn into creative solutions. Give up black-and-white thinking—

right *or* wrong, good *vs.* bad. There are many ways to skin a cat. Maybe your mistake will help you find a new one.

10. When problems do occur, focus on teamwork effectiveness rather than individual blame. Punishment leads to stress, even for the punisher. A teamwork approach focuses on what can be learned and how to avoid the problem in the future.

OVERVIEW OF A STRESS-FREE LIFE

In this chapter, we've covered the gamut of stress reduction, from meditation at home to focusing on teamwork at the office. You might feel stressed merely at the thought of remembering all this information. So in keeping with our stress-free approach to life, here's an overview that will help you put it all together.

1. Call a halt to the madness.
   - give yourself time to enjoy the simple pleasures of life
   - reconnect with your inner self
   - allow your creative self to emerge

2. Avoid myths about "being a man" that create more stress.

3. Replace anger with constructive communication.
   - take responsibility for your actions instead of blaming others
   - make sure you hear one another before lashing out
   - have "pow-wows" before tensions build too high

4. Enjoy your family.
   - have a vote on family matters
   - develop family rituals
     • create special messages that can be sent by digital pager
     • have a family brunch or dinner every Sunday
     • read the Sunday paper together, sharing comics, puzzles, spórts, and so on.

5. Reduce stress at work.

6. Allow yourself "escape" techniques once in a while.

7. Acquire good sleeping habits.

8. Learn meditation and yoga techniques to help your body remain youthful.

— CHART I —
STEPS TO DEALING WITH CONFLICT

When:	What:
Before arguing	Know what you want
You express your opinion	Don't blame
You're ready to respond to your partner's statement	Make sure you've heard what's been said
You specify what change you want	Explain how it affects you
Arguing becomes too intense	Use "T" sign for time out
At all times	Use common courtesy and respect
Next time	Plan regular discussions to prevent conflict

— CHART II —
HOW STRESS AFFECTS YOUR BODY

Head	Tension headaches, forgetfulness, inability to concentrate
Ears	Ringing
Shoulders	Hunching over, as in "I feel like I've got the weight of the world on my shoulders."
Chest	Racing heart, high blood pressure, palpitations

Stomach	Cramps, heartburn, indigestion
Back	Lower back pains due to spasms
Genitals	Lower sex drive

KEEPING YOUR
SEXUALITY YOUNG AND
STRONG

CHAPTER 4

"I feel like a million bucks," claimed 77-year-old Dean Martin, as he began to celebrate New Year's Eve this year. Accompanied by his ex-wife Jeanne and friend Ursula Andress at a posh Beverly Hills restaurant, Dean was seen as fit, in great spirits and happy to be alive. "What a great new year it's going to be," he told reporters, before getting into his Rolls-Royce. "I can't wait!"

Dean Martin has been a sex idol most of his adult life. And even into his 70s, almost pushing 80, he manages to still carry it off successfully.

As we look forward to ten more years of healthy life, can we also anticipate them as sexy years? What is the real truth on male sexuality as we mature? What role does sex play in enhancing a more youthful life?

Why not ask actor Anthony Quinn who fathered his eleventh child at the age of 78? Or you might want to confer with Tom Temple (not his real name), one of my patients.

After 50 years of marriage, 85-year-old Tom Temple is still enjoying daily sex with his wife. Both he and his wife are now retired and enjoying one another's company on their small farm in Georgia. Tom creates wooden toys in his workshop in his spare time but whenever he's near his wife, the affection he showers on her can be seen quite clearly. Both Tom and his wife look significantly younger than their years. Does their ongoing sexual involvement help keep them young?

HOW TO PROLONG YOUR SEX LIFE

According to a study done at the Royal Edinburgh Hospital in Scotland, people who looked an average of 15 years younger than their peers had at least this in common: They tended to have sex on a daily basis.

Check with Your Partner First

But before you run for the bedroom with unrealistic expectations, you should know the following: Almost all couples disagree about how frequently they "should" have sex. Furthermore, for most couples, there is a definite and distinct decrease in the frequency and intensity of sex after marriage.

Unequal Sex Drives

During courtship, we put our best foot forward not only in terms of appearance, courtesy, and devotion, but also in terms of our sexuality. We're eager to please in all areas, including sex. After the wedding, when we've already been "captured" by our mate, the pretenses disappear and reality takes over. Sexual needs are now expressed more realistically. Usually, one partner has a stronger sex drive than the other. This may take a few months or years to be revealed, but that day (or night) may finally come when a healthy sexual appetite may be frustrated as a spouse begins to fall back on suspicious "headaches," as in "Not tonight, dear. . . ."

Courtship can be as different from marriage as packaging is from contents. What you see initially is supposed to advertise what follows, but "truth in advertising," considered an oxymoron by many, is not always dependable.

Many of my patients have complained of a pattern in which sexual attraction for one or the other of the partners declines drastically immediately following the wedding. As we explored the reasons, all we could come up with was the difference between pursuing a partner during courtship and distancing a partner after marriage in order to conserve a certain amount of "breathing space" to counteract the accommodations and sacrifices necessary to make a marriage work. At this point the party with the lower sex drive will initiate the distancing, making the other party feel the crush of rejection.

Tony and Amanda, working together in their home-based computer company, were married only six months, but they already had sexual differences between them. Amanda had a rich sexual history prior to meeting Tony. She had to have sex at least on a weekly basis, whether or not she had a regular boyfriend at the time. But soon after the wedding it was Tony who was making more sexual demands, while Amanda's drive seemed almost to disappear.

The more Tony pushed, the less interested Amanda became. The conflict and tension between them increased dramatically. Apparently, Amanda was feeling that her independence and "personal space" were being threatened. Their working together in the family business also didn't help matters. As with many similar couples, the more Tony pushed, the more Amanda pulled away. The chasm between the two constantly feuding partners was becoming impassable.

A vicious cycle may begin in which the disparity between the two levels of sex drive becomes greater and greater. The "pursuer" becomes more insecure and needy while the "pursued" becomes less tolerant of the pursuing partner's insecurities. The not-tonight-dear "headache" may start very soon after the wedding but that is rare. More likely, it will take months or years for the "pursued" to take action in the form of excuses.

Different Strokes for Different Folks

This shouldn't come as any surprise. We all differ in so many respects—energy level, curiosity, need for social involvement, appetite for food—why not appetite for sex! There is probably a widespread misconception that couples who are happily married should have similar sexual desires over the years. Sometimes this happens, sometimes it doesn't.

Learn to Negotiate

Rather than becoming a source of stress, tension over when to have sex can be overcome by good communication. To ensure a stress-free sexual relationship, the couple must learn to negotiate—not only about frequency, but also about other facets of sexuality. I suggested to Tony and Amanda that they make "sex dates" for times when neither was too busy or too tired, and to plan for variety in sex.

This approach gave both partners a sense of control over their own lives, instead of Tony feeling rejected and Amanda feeling pushed. By planning for variety, both had the opportunity for give and take in offering and receiving from one another. This encouraged them to communicate more freely about what turned each of them on. This way Amanda had more to look forward to, as did Tony, of course. The pressure to perform was replaced with an invitation to dialogue and explore.

Whatever Turns You On

According to Steven Carter and Julia Sokol, authors of *What Really Happens in Bed*, some people love oral sex, others hate it; some like fantasy role-playing, others are turned off by it; some like to talk in bed, others find it distracting; some enjoy acrobatic sex, others prefer a single position.

The Real Truth About Sex

According to these authors, most of us harbor sexual myths that can create unwarranted stress in our relationships:

1. *Myth*: Good sex should be spontaneous.

   Truth: Spontaneity is neither realistic nor always desirable. Planning ahead allows for anticipation, preparation, and mood-setting.

2. *Myth*: Great sex equals a great relationship.

   Truth: The most unhappy couples can be having great sex. Conversely, strong, loving marriages survive sexual challenges. What really keeps a relationship going strong are commitment, love, and mutual respect.

3. *Myth*: Simultaneous orgasm is the ideal.

   Truth: Not so! Sexual satisfaction has little to do with this.

4. *Myth*: Women should have multiple orgasms.

Truth: Many women reported that they did not always need to have an orgasm to find sex very pleasurable. And no one (man or woman) likes to be pressured to climax. (It is important, however, for both partners to put the extra effort into ensuring an orgasm for the woman, at least occasionally.)

5. *Myth*: The longer men can hold out, the better.

Truth: Partially so. But many maturing couples made the surprising report that men with serious erection problems can be the most satisfying lovers. The key for these couples was to shift the focus to erotic experiences surrounding intercourse.

Seventy to eighty percent of men and women over 50, for example, enjoy sexual arousal by stimulation of the woman's breasts and nipples. Manual stimulation of one another's genitals continues to be a source of pleasure for couples well into their 70s and 80s, despite erection difficulties. Stroking of the penis can restore potency in many elderly men and, even when it doesn't, mutual stroking of penis and clitoris can be quite satisfying. An 80-year-old couple refers to this as "a very pleasant supplement to intercourse."

Since true intimacy is an important component in adding ten years of youthful life, it's essential to keep sex from creating distance between the members of a couple. One way of overcoming this distance between men and women in romantic relationships is to reveal the following five sexual secrets in order to "demythify" the sexes from one another.

FIVE SECRETS ABOUT SEX

First Secret: Just about everyone masturbates, regardless of age, marital status, religious affiliation, or social status. By the way, it does not cause blindness.

Second Secret: Although having sexual fantasies can be great, acting them out is most often disappointing. This is a case in which anticipation is much greater than the realization. The best sex is based on reality, genuine love, and honest communication. Loving honesty and self-revelation are the best aphrodisiacs. Within such a relationship, there's no need to pay for a trip to Hawaii to enjoy a moonlit night on the beach. Get comfortable in your own bedroom, let your minds wander, and let your "fingers do the walking." You can make love under the stars and pretend it's Hawaii, or in the shower, pretending you're under a waterfall.

Third Secret: All men have sexual anxieties at one time or another. Of course, this increases as we get older. A man's penis is not a piece of plumbing—it's an integral part of his person. And if things aren't going right in his mind or heart, then his penis will not be right as well. Women who don't realize this may put tremendous pressure on men to perform. But when heart and mind are connected in a good, loving relationship, there are always ways to overcome any sexual challenge.

One technique that works very well to persuade a reluctant penis is for your woman to try the following technique: Teach her to stroke, gently and slowly, the shaft of the penis in one hand with a gentle up and down motion while lightly massaging the head of the penis with the palm of the other hand. As the penis begins to respond, she can continue the slow, unhurried pace until you are fully aroused.

Fourth Secret: Almost all women have faked orgasm. Just as there is pressure on us to perform, so is there pressure on women. Only women can fake it, whereas we men cannot even fake erection. Since women's orgasms are likewise connected to their hearts and minds, orgasms aren't always forthcoming. At such times, faking it can be a much simpler option than creating a sense of frustration, disappointment, and possibly a fight. Sometimes faking it is okay, but even better is honest communication, support, and accepting that the holding and tenderness are what are really important. As a couple develops a strong level of honesty and acceptance of one another, faking orgasms is no longer necessary.

Fifth Secret: Most men and women in relationships keep their sexual secrets from one another. Typically, in most relationships, sexual development takes place much more quickly than emotional disclosure. Another way to put it: Men and women take their clothes off more quickly than they bare their souls. And so, in those relationships that last, sexual patterns tend to set in before sexual idiosyncrasies have a chance to be discussed. Once the sexual patterns are set, it becomes even more difficult to discuss changes, because we sense our own and each other's sexual vulnerabilities so keenly.

Discuss Sex Honestly

There's one simple solution to all problems arising out of these five sexual secrets: better communication. Couples that can take the time and energy to discuss deep emotional and sexual issues (it's amazing how these go together) will benefit greatly in terms of opening up possibilities of loving communication and support. Reevaluating sexual needs and tastes can help greatly. If it doesn't come easily, then consider counseling, or support groups, or a trip to the library to read up on it. To the extent that life is short (although ten years longer if we do it right), then it's worthwhile to take the plunge into more honest sexual discussion to make the rest of our lives (plus ten years) happier.

How to Approach the Subject of Sex

Here are some helpful hints on how to get down to the nitty-gritty discussion about sex with your lover. First, pick the right time. Actually make a date for this important discussion. Say something like, "Honey, when you have time I've got something really important that I'd like to talk about." Make sure you listen to one another, rather than lecture your partner. Sometimes we need to stop and let the other person talk.

Our Deeper Sexual Needs

When our deeper sexual needs are revealed and discussed openly, we really end up showing how much we need to feel loved and accepted in an emotional/social sense. Once these deeper needs are accepted and attention paid to them, it's amazing how the remaining problems in our life become so easily dealt with.

SO MUCH FOR FOREPLAY: NOW ABOUT SEX!

But first this news from the latest Kinsey Report on Sex:

"Most women prefer a sexual partner who has a large penis."
"Sex usually ends soon after age 60."
"Masturbation is physically harmful."
"Most normal women have orgasms from penile thrusting alone."
"A man cannot have an orgasm without an erection."

—Time Magazine

This quotation from *Time* magazine came from an article describing the latest Kinsey Report. But you should know the heading above the quotes:

"All Wrong: Myths About Sex"

According to the Kinsey Report, of all 2,000 subjects polled, only slightly over half responded correctly to questions about sexuality. Many believed the above-quoted myths to be true.

In fact, some women like large penises, but most are more concerned with the "motion of the ocean" rather than the "size of the ship."

In fact, masturbation does *not* lead to blindness or even to needing glasses. It can be a very important component of a healthy sex life, especially for those not in a stable romantic or married relationship (not that they're exclusive). It can be important for the sex lives of married people as well.

In fact, many women achieve orgasm not from penile thrusting alone, but rather from manual, oral or even mechanical (as in vibrator) stimulation. There's nothing wrong with any of this. I can't help but say it: Different strokes for different folks.

In fact, it is possible for men to achieve orgasm without an erection.

Now, here's the most important one of all!

In fact, sex does *not* usually end soon after age 60. It lasts throughout our lives, even into the additional ten years. Each decade of life can bring greater sexual satisfaction. Here's how.

In their 30s, men begin to find release from their preoccupation with orgasms and many women begin to experience orgasm for the very first time. So an opportunity for sexual mutuality becomes available for the first time.

In their 40s, men become more sensual and less obsessive about sex. Women become more confident about their sexuality as men open up to their sexual vulnerability. The result—less emphasis on quick sex and greater opportunities for sensuality, creative foreplay, and longer lasting sex.

In their 50s, women begin shifting into high gear, sexually speaking. As their estrogen levels drop, they're more responsive to the sexually driven androgens in their bodies. Since men's erections are now less spontaneous—though 98 percent are still sexually active—both enjoy the more extended time for sensual foreplay and creative sexuality.

In their 60s, 91 percent of men are still sexually active, though erectile fullness may decrease for some men and vaginal lubrication may decrease for some women. But sexual satisfaction need not decrease. Morning erections can still be counted on, so timing can take care of the man's problem.

In their 70s, 80 percent are still interested in sex and 70 percent are having sex about once a week. Playful and sexual massage becomes a more integral part of the sex as men may enjoy up to 30 to 40 minutes of foreplay to become fully erect. No complaints from the women on that score. There is now more time to relax—no pressures or distractions from crying babies or demanding teenagers—so there's the luxury of affording themselves more tenderness and gentleness.

In their 80s, during the ten extra years, sex can get even better. According to a survey of 800 elderly couples, women still have the capacity for orgasms, and 50 percent of men in their 80s are still interested in sex and can still have erections. Now here's the clincher: 75 percent of those who are still sexually active say that their lovemaking has actually improved!

A recent sex survey published this past year by the University of Chicago reveals that Americans are more monogamous than we ever imagined, and that married couples have the best sex at least twice a week or more. The survey also revealed that nearly 75 percent of married men are faithful to their wives and most enjoy watching their partners undress. According to the authors, "married people are all alike—they are faithful to their partners as long as the marriage is intact."

As Garrison Keillor, of A *Prairie Home Companion* fame, puts it: "It is almost worth all the misery of dealing with real estate people, bankers, lawyers, and contractors—to have a home that has a bedroom where the two of you can go sometimes and do this. It is worth growing up and becoming middle-aged to be able to enjoy it utterly."

At the same time, a second sexual revolution has recently taken place, according to the recent Janus Report on sexual behavior, characterized in part by "a regeneration of sexual interest and behavior among the postmature population." For example, about one in seven men over the age of 65 still enjoy sexual activity on a daily basis, and all adults are more experimental than ever in their approaches to sexuality.

Men up to age 90, according to the report, continue to have sex as long as they have a partner in whom they're interested and report finding their sexual experience "as gratifying as ever." Men stay just as sexually active into their 60s (81 percent) as they were in their 30s (83 percent) and 40s (83 percent). After age 65, 69 percent of men continue to have sex at least once a week. The ability of these men over age 65 to "have 'functionally' successful sex diminished very little from their earlier years," according to the report. So, all in all, as you look forward to ten extra years of healthy life, you can also anticipate a vigorous, fun-filled sex life during those years.

SIX WAYS TO STAY YOUNG SEXUALLY

In the past few years there has been a hubbub of interest in the possibility of sex-enhancing drugs. My own feeling is that if any of these drugs worked perfectly, the media would be all over them and such successful drugs would become the fashion of the day. Nonetheless, a number of these drugs have proven at least partially successful if we can believe the scientists' research results as well as the anecdotal accounts of some satisfied users. So let's at least look at the best of these drugs, starting with the most familiar—coffee!

1. Coffee Can Be Sexy

Although scientists can't explain the process, it appears that drinking coffee can enhance your sex drive. At the University of Michigan, researchers found that, of 744 coffee-drinking, married couples over the age of 60, 62 percent described themselves as "sexually active" as compared with 38 percent of non-coffee drinkers. The men who were coffee drinkers also reported fewer erection problems.

2. Yohimbine Strengthens Erections

Hundreds of years ago European sailors returning from Africa brought back a substance from the bark of an African tree. Known as yohimbine, this substance was used as an aphrodisiac. To test the effectiveness of this potion, scientists at Stanford University injected this substance into two groups of rats—one normal group and one impotent group. Following the injections the normal rats mounted females at twice the normal rate, while half the formerly impotent rats began mating.

At Queens University Hospital in Canada, a doctor tried this potion on humans. He gave 6 mg. of this substance three times a day to 23 impotent men. Ten of them were helped by the drug and six reported full erections and full sexual function.

Yohimbine works in part by enhancing stimulation of the sympathetic nervous system, which encourages an erection. At this point, yohimbine continues to facilitate the sympathetic nervous system, resulting in increased sexual desire and pleasure. Although yohimbine doesn't work for all men, it's worth a try if your physician agrees. It is a prescription medication.

3. Levodopa and Eldepryl Boost the Sex Urge

Somewhat less effective, but nonetheless that stand out above the crowd of supposed sex-enhancing drugs, are two that deserve our attention: Levodopa (or L-dopa) and deprenyl (or Eldepryl). Both require a prescription, and both take several weeks to work.

Both work in a similar fashion. You see, as we age, the neurotransmitter dopamine decreases in our body. This important chemical transmits brain messages and is important to sex drive, among other functions. These two sex-enhancing drugs both affect the dopamine levels in the brain.

Levodopa is an amino acid that increases the levels of dopamine in the brain, resulting in an emotional high and a temporary boost to the sexual urge. Both drugs end up increasing the amount of dopamine, although their routes are different.

Eldepryl is a relatively safe drug. One of its benefits is that it not only maintains higher, healthier levels of dopamine, it also appears to keep the dopamine-producing cells from deteriorating with age. The dosage for Eldepryl as a sex-enhancing drug can range from 5 mg. twice a week to 5 mg./day, depending on your age and how quickly you respond to it. In any case, you'll have to work with your doctor to find the dosage that best suits you. When it does work, the effects can be quite dramatic. Or it may not work for you at all. But it's certainly worth a try if other approaches haven't worked.

4. Phentolamine—Produces Erections

The prospect of living and loving ten years longer could never have come at a better time. For some of you, the above-mentioned suggestions will suffice; others may need more. But as time goes by, more and more options become available. For example, in the late 1980s, one company successfully experimented with a new drug, *quinelorane*, which could stimulate the brain's dopamine receptors, thereby intensifying arousal.

The experiment to test the effectiveness of the drug involved over 500 individuals from 15 major medical centers across the country. The drug appeared to be effective for women and at least some men, but it had the unfortunate side effect of producing nausea. So the research for quinelorane stopped for the time being. But who knows what's around the corner! As I write, it's rumored that two pharmaceutical companies are working on sex enhancers. It's only a matter of time. And, if we continue to do things right, we've got ten years more to enjoy them all.

Another promising drug that has been successful in the injection form is now being considered as an oral drug. Dr. Adrian Zorgniotti, Professor of Clinical Urology at New York University, used the drug phentolamine in 50 mg. capsules on 100 impotent patients. In the first experiments reported at the Annual Meeting of the American Urological Association, the doctor prescribed sexual inter-course two hours after giving 85 of his impotent patients the 50 mg. capsules. Forty-two percent were able to achieve full erections and an additional 18 percent were able to achieve partial erections.

This was successful enough to attempt to fine tune the proce-dure. Next, the doctor had 31 of his patients place a smaller tablet, 20 mg. this time, between the gum and cheek. This route allowed quick-er absorption of the pill and so the patients attempted intercourse after only 20 minutes. Lo and behold—almost half of them were able to attain full erections and another 5 achieved partial erections.

5. The Bean Connection

If you want to try the non-prescription route, you can try fava beans, which have a high concentration of levodopa. A 16-ounce can of these beans practically offers a prescription dose. If it works for you, great! If not, at least you've had a healthy, fiber-filled meal.

6. Alcohol Doesn't Help

First, let's review the physical factors. If you follow the guidelines later on in this book—stopping smoking, getting your exercise, eat-ing healthfully and taking your vitamin supplements—then your body should be in excellent shape. One topic I've chosen not to deal with in this book is alcoholism, but mention needs to be made here that alcohol consumption can lower potency both in the short run (a few drinks may hamper the ability to achieve an erection) as well as in the long run (heavy drinking can eventually damage the nerves that trigger an erection).

(Although I've chosen not to focus on alcohol as a factor in longevity, I can confidently say that the bottom-line solution to an alcohol problem consists of only two letters: A.A. Alcoholics Anonymous is by far the best solution. Resistance to this solution is almost always defensive rationalizing. So what's the point of saying any more on this topic!)

OVERCOMING IMPOTENCE

Although most men experience changes in their sex drive as the years go by, this "inevitable decline" does not necessarily mean that you can't go on enjoying a fully satisfying sex life even as you live ten years longer. As long as you stay healthy and fit, enjoyable sex can go on and on.

Of course, as time goes by, you may become more susceptible to factors contributing to occasions where erection does not come as easily as it has in the past. We'll discuss these factors shortly, but be assured that occasional "problems" are normal. They *don't* mean an inevitable slide into permanent impotence.

A little alcohol, for example, may be relaxing, but too much can be debilitating. More trouble may be caused by a medication you're currently taking. Different medications have different effects on different people.

Some men fear a smaller penis may contribute to problems of impotence. Not so! The same physiology is part of a small penis as a large penis—no difference as far as susceptibility to impotence. And fears that too much masturbation will lead to impotence are also totally unfounded.

What *is* true is that as a man ages the time elapsed before he can get aroused again becomes greater. No more three-times-in-a-row as you mature. As time goes by, you may need to wait until the next night to become aroused again.

What is also true is that it'll take longer for you to get aroused as you mature. Middle-aged men take almost six times longer to get aroused than those in their 20s. Their erections may be slightly less firm and their ejaculations less forceful. However, precisely because there is less urgency, middle-aged men can more likely relax and more fully enjoy their sexual encounters.

Almost all men, regardless of age, have, at one time or another, experienced some difficulty maintaining an erection. In this chapter, we'll explore the major causes of such problems and discuss how to keep your sex organs young and strong.

CAUSES OF IMPOTENCE

Dan, a teacher, and Mary, a social worker, both in their 40s, cared for one another deeply, but her sex drive was greater than his. Mary was getting discouraged after hearing an ongoing sequence of "Not tonight, dear," responses to her affectionate overtures. Like many other couples, Mary and Dan had different appetites for sex.

When I interviewed Dan alone in my office, it turned out there were a number of factors affecting his sex drive, though he was quite unaware of this. Although he definitely was not what anyone would consider an alcoholic, Dan occasionally enjoyed a couple of glasses of wine during dinner, and perhaps an additional glass after dinner on Saturdays when he could stay up later than usual. Also, although Dan was far from a chronic smoker, he'd light up a few following Saturday's dinner for the same reason. This was *his* evening, to be fully enjoyed, especially since this was when he and Mary typically made love, or at least tried to.

Dan confided in me that he feared he was becoming impotent. As we talked further, it became clear that there were other factors as well. Dan had recently discovered that his blood pressure was borderline high, possibly due to the increasing pressures he felt at school, where more and more paperwork was being demanded of him. As a result, his family doctor had prescribed a tranquilizer and a popular hypertension medication.

Dan had confused feelings about all this. He was angry at the prospect of having to take medication, since he prided himself on his successful attempts at staying fit and healthy till this recent diagnosis. He was also frustrated at not being able to please Mary in bed. We soon both came to the conclusion that all this came close to a classic case of "performance anxiety," especially since Mary had been sharing with Dan the stories her girlfriends told her about their exploits with their super-stud lovers. Contributing to the performance anxiety was a developing case of "great expectations." Dan was on the verge of becoming depressed, unless I could help him with his problem. (Dan's story continues on page 97.)

Dan's case is one that reflects many of the problems experienced by men suffering from impotence. Impotence is defined as difficulty in achieving or maintaining an erection. It used to be thought that virtually all such problems were "in the head." Now we realize that half the problem is physical. But let's start by looking at what's "in the head."

Psychological/Emotional Factors

1. *Performance anxiety.* This can occur for any activity. Authors get writer's block. Baseball players get into slumps and public performers get stage fright. So it shouldn't come as a surprise that occasionally men become blocked, go into a slump, or get frightened about their sexual performance. This is normal. What is not normal is when this anxiety begins to persist and feeds on itself so that the man feels totally inadequate as a sexual partner and his sex life goes down the drain for long periods of time. Each failed attempt reinforces his sense of sexual inadequacy. When more than one in four attempts end in failure, we have a full-blown case of impotence, caused by performance anxiety.

2. *Great expectations.* Another cause of sexual stress is the pressure put on men by accounts of super-sex in the media. Typically, more and more movies contain at least one torrid sex scene to make sure they're competitive at the box office. Men see their heroes erotically ravish their partners on kitchen sinks (*Fatal Attraction*) on the subway (*Speed*), on the piano (*Pretty Woman*), while playing the piano (*The Piano*), underwater and in the air (James Bond), and so on, with such romantic passion that they begin to feel inadequate about their human limitations.

3. *Life's hard knocks.* As men mature, life usually becomes more and more challenging, with increasing responsibilities. Families become larger and more complex, what with children marrying and divorcing, not to mention their own divorces. Financial responsibilities increase in the form of increased mortgages and loan balances; job responsibilities increase as they climb the career ladder. For those marriages that survive, there's a spouse with her own life changes to deal with, possibly leading to more misunderstandings and arguments.

The increasing number of deaths and illnesses among friends and acquaintances, changes in their own health, midlife repositioning, seeing younger men come up to compete for their positions at work, inevitable legal hassles, an increasing professional liability, poor investment risks they took on at an earlier age, or problems brought on by misdeeds of their offspring all lead to an increasing sense of pressure as midlife approaches. Then they expect themselves to plop into bed at night and instantly become the James Bond of their bedroom. Unrealistic? You bet!

4. *The influence of personality*

   a. Mr. *Independence* avoids rejection by accepting as little as possible from the women in his life. His relationships are characterized by promiscuity rather than commitment, more detachment than intimacy. He takes major pride in his independent stance.

      The problem is that as he matures, total independence no longer works. His increasing vulnerability, both physically as well as socially and emotionally, creates an impasse. The loss of his prized independence creates a great deal of anxiety and a reexamination of his values. One possible result: a full-blown case of impotence.

   b. Mr. *Pleaser* aims to please everyone but himself. He's made happy when all around him are happy. He takes pride in his ability to please others, even when his own needs are totally ignored. Most important is that everyone likes him, which is the source of his self-esteem.

      Women love Mr. Pleaser, and why not! He does all he can to make sure their sexual experiences are great. Only problem is that as he matures, Mr. Pleaser begins to wane in his physical prowess and no longer has such a strong emotional base from which to please his women, as much as he aspires. One possible result: a stressful case of performance anxiety.

   c. Mr. *Success* can do it all, earlier and better than other men. He creates risk in his life and plays to win, with a strong belief that once he achieves his dreams, his insecurities will vanish. He steps around, over, and even on others to further his progress. In the bedroom, he's a master of technique, taking pride in how well he manipulates a woman to orgasm.

With age, Mr. Success may lose his edge not only in the board room, but in the bedroom as well. The Nobel prize has evaded his grasp, and so has the heart of any special woman. Lacking in any semblance of human warmth and human kindness, sex becomes more and more of a drag for him. Women find younger men more attractive and Mr. Success is losing it to the point where this self-induced pressure may lead to—you guessed it—a full-blown case of impotence.

d. Mr. Mad is an angry young man at the start, taking pride in his ability to intimidate all those around him. His ability to control others gives him a strong sense of inner strength. Disagree with him and you incur his wrath.

In his youth, Mr. Mad may intimidate women into complying with his sexual demands and he enjoys his dominating rule. But as he matures, his intimidating style becomes more and more empty, lacking any semblance of human warmth. When most men begin to enjoy the sensual and emotional aspects of sex, he is left high and dry in the loneliness of his angry world. His angry feelings make erotic arousal more and more difficult—another case of full-blown impotence.

e. Finally, we present Mr. Helper, the professional guru who has answers for all those prepared to pay his fees. He has a genuine interest in helping people so long as they come to his office and defer to his status as a professional helper. His sense of commitment is to the outside world, with little time left for those closest to him. Having dedicated his youth to graduate education, he tends to pamper himself with adult toys (cars, sound systems, exotic travel) which leave him even less time for real intimacy with loved ones.

The result is inevitable. The outside world is so involving and seductive that his heart and soul have little energy left for meaningful communication with those closest to him. When he gets home, the meter is turned off and he withdraws to inner contemplation or superficial recreation. Becoming vulnerable with intimacy would destroy the sense of super-competence associated with his professional status. For Mr. Helper, it is not so much a case of sexual failure as much as sexual disinterest. Yet the bottom line is sexual incompleteness, a kind of impotence by occupational hazard.

5. *Depression*. There are two types of depression—one that follows a traumatic event, and one that occurs for no obvious reason, except for the ongoing onslaught of life's general, increasing pressures. In either case, the depressed individual has a general sense of unworthiness. He sleeps poorly if at all, loses his appetite for food, music, and even sex. This, however, is not the same as impotence, since attaining and maintaining erections is not difficult. The depressed man can engage in sex—it's just that his sex drive is very low.

6. *Boredom*. After many years of marriage, the ongoing familiarity of the same sex partner, the same lovemaking patterns and the same setting may eventually take a toll. When this ongoing sameness is paired with a gradual reduction in sex drive in the context of increasing pressures of responsibility, a form of psychological impotence can occur. There is essentially nothing wrong with the individual, either physiologically or emotionally, but this deadly combination of patterns may result in a lack of sexual interest in many ways akin to impotence.

Physical Factors

1. *Toxic impotence*. A number of medications have been implicated in contributing to causing and abetting impotence, particularly those used to counteract high blood pressure. The difficulty in isolating the "guilty" drugs lies in the fact that all drugs affect men differently as far as their contribution to the impotence problem. Furthermore, the same man may be affected by a certain drug at one point in his life and not in another. To complicate things even further, two drugs taken separately may have no effect on a certain individual, but may have a very damaging effect when taken together.

Blood pressure medicines and diuretics (for example *Diuril*, *Catapres*, *Lopressor*) are the most culpable, but other classes of drugs such as tranquilizers (such as *Thorazine*, *Mellaril*, *Prolixin*), antidepressants (for example *Elavil*, *Tofranil*, *Sinequan*), antihistamines (for example, *Benadryl*), and muscle relaxants (such as *Flexeril*) can also contribute to impotence. Even other drugs such as *Dilantin* (for seizures), *Flagyl* (for infections), and *Tagamet* (for ulcers) can get in on the act.

It's not clear whether these drugs act directly to inhibit the sex centers of the brain or interfere with the nerves relating to erection physiology.

2. *Smoking*. Smoking can affect potency in two ways. First, since smoking tends to have the effect of hardening and narrowing the arteries in general, it also has the same effect locally in the penis.

Second, in about 5 percent of men, an extreme sensitivity to smoke exists, causing a marked constriction of the blood vessels leading to the chambers of the penis involved in erection. Fortunately, these effects are reversible when smoking is given up.

3. *Alcohol*. As for the effect of alcohol on potency, Shakespeare said it best: "It provokes the desire, but it takes away the performance." Put in modern terms, alcohol reduces inhibitions, but it also tends to depress many brain functions as well as the sexual response. An initial bout of impotence due to alcohol can sometimes be the first step in creating a fear which, over time, may result in full-blown performance anxiety.

Beyond the temporary effects of alcohol are the long-lasting effects of chronic alcoholism. The effect on the body is two-fold: first, it can interfere with the testicles' ability to produce testosterone, and second, it can affect the liver so as to change the way the body uses whatever testosterone *is* produced. For those who give up alcohol, about half will regain normal potency but unfortunately half will not.

In a small number of men, potency is enhanced by alcohol and is absent during sobriety. This may be because in such men psychological inhibitions to sex are a greater problem than is physiology. For such men, this creates quite a dilemma. In the long run, however, potency may be adversely affected by alcohol.

SOLUTIONS TO IMPOTENCE

As Dan sat across from me in my office, the late afternoon sun's rays cutting through the window blinds, I began to develop a program to save him from impending depression. I knew how proud he was of his physique and degree of fitness, given his fortysomething age. I knew how he felt a loss of independence, being relegated to daily pills for his anxiety and moderate blood pressure.

"Dan," I asked, "how often do you work out these days?"

"Not like I used to," he replied. "That darn paperwork has taken up so much of my time. I've even had to give up my meditation and little bit of yoga that I used to do."

"OK, I've got the answer," I finally decided. "Here's what I recommend. Let me talk to Dr. Lewison and discuss the possibility of you going off the medicines he prescribed if you'll agree to resume your jogging and meditation, and if you'll let me work with you on quitting smoking and easing up on your wine quota."

"You've got a deal," Dan beamed happily. And we spent our remaining time discussing the rest of the solution: How to deal with the difference in appetite between him and Mary.

First of all, I told him, pleasing Mary did not include competing with her girlfriends' lovers. From what Dan shared with me, Mary was more than content with Dan's sexual style, if only he could "get it up." Why not make this a part of sex play! If Dan could encourage Mary to try more foreplay, including oral and manual stimulation, then the problem, along with the other measures we were incorporating, would most likely be solved.

"But," interjected Dan, "sometimes I'm just not in the mood. I don't want to have to perform on a routine basis, as if I were a machine! How can I let Mary know that without hurting her feelings?"

"Simple," I responded. "Mary is quite reasonable and understanding. Why don't you negotiate the following? Give her some kind of signal to let her know when you're in the mood. . .something simple." I thought for a moment as Dan glanced at his watch. "That's it! If you're in the mood when you go to bed at night, just leave your wristwatch on. That'll be the signal to Mary that you're open to being turned on. When you take off your wristwatch, she'll understand you're not in the mood."

"Great, Doc," said Dan, beaming with satisfaction, "that way we won't even have to talk about it if I'm not in the mood." Dan and Mary's problems were solved. The impending problem of impotence had been solved!

What *not* to do is to ignore the problem of impotence. Many men shy away from confronting the issue by actively ignoring it. This will not solve the problem. Unfortunately, in our culture many men equate their self-worth to their sexual prowess.

The first step in dealing with the problem is to determine whether it really exists or not. If it does exist, the next step is to determine whether the cause is more likely physical or psychological. Here's a brief test to help you determine that. Just circle the appropriate number and then add up all your circled numbers.

PHYSICAL IMPOTENCE INVENTORY

	True	?	False
1. My overall health is good.	3	2	1
2. I tend to overuse alcohol or drugs.	1	2	3
3. I'm taking medication.	1	2	3
4. I have suffered a groin injury.	1	2	3
5. At times, I awake with morning erections.	3	2	1
6. During masturbation, full erection is sustained until climax.	3	2	1
7. My sexual appetite hasn't changed.	3	2	1

Scores over 17 indicate a greater likelihood of psychological impotence or no impotence at all. Scores under 17 indicate a greater likelihood of physical impotence. In this case consult with your physician.

Sex Therapy

If you scored over 18 and you are suffering from impotence, you're a likely candidate for sex therapy. The main thing is to find a competent professional or institute. Individual sex therapists should be certified by the American Association of Sex Educators, Counselors and Therapists, and be licensed to practice in your state. Other therapists dealing with potency problems should likewise be licensed by the state in which they practice. Always inquire about such matters.

A competent sex therapist will most likely interview you in depth about your medical, personal, and sexual history and discuss your expectations from such therapy.

Some therapists may explore the use of *sensate focus*, as developed by Masters and Johnson. This involves trying out new patterns of sexual stimulation and enhanced communication between you and your partner. A certain amount of discipline and guided structure is involved, which aims for open communication and sensitive yet respectful sexual stimulation between the two of you. Currently, there is a growing library of educational videotapes to complement such programs. Generally, the aim is to enhance sexual pleasure while keeping any anxiety about performance as low as possible.

Self-help

Because of this burgeoning industry of videotape sex education and many more books on the topic, it's possible to avoid paying the expense of a professional and select the materials you're most comfortable with. If this fails, you can always fall back on a professional.

If you choose the self-help option, here are some guidelines:

1. Maintain open communication between you and your partner about what feels good for either of you.

   You might even communicate without words. One way you can communicate with your lover exactly what you want in foreplay is to guide the hand that caresses you. If a picture is worth a thousand words, certainly a little guidance in the right direction is worth at least a hundred.

2. Another helpful suggestion to keep sex dynamic is to share the initiative in sexual play. Give each partner a chance to have a different role—being the active or the passive one. The most dynamic sex involves a mutual give and take between partners. That's what helps keep sex from becoming boring over the years.

Learn to reverse roles in terms of initiative, dominance, pleasuring. Take turns in terms of who takes responsibility for the sexual encounter, who takes charge while being sexual and who gives rather than receives more stimulation.

Just as men and women have both male and female qualities embedded within their deeper selves, so do both enjoy the dominant and submissive roles at different times. It's fun to allow each role to come to the fore as it emerges naturally, driven by sexual desire. As the more dominant partner takes the risk of allowing the other to take over, trust between the two has a chance to grow. Risk-taking at the horizontal level has a chance to spill over into the vertical level. Good sex can contribute to improving the marriage.

3. Pick a time and a place that is comfortable and free from distraction. If you can't get away for the weekend, at least turn off the phone and send the kids to a movie.

   Selecting time for sex is also important. Weekend mornings are a good time. Or afternoons. Or in the early evening. . . don't save the lovemaking until you're exhausted. The point is: Give sex the priority it deserves! Consider it a date in the same way you make dates to do other things. Create an atmosphere beforehand with candles and wine and whatever it is that makes you feel that it's special. Occasionally creating some kind of ambience satisfies the need to be romantic. You'd be surprised how few people do that.

4. Make sure you and your partner are feeling good about one another. Don't try to patch up a bad argument by having sex. It won't work, at least for most people.

5. This may be obvious to most, but make sure you're both clean and smelling fresh and pleasant. Have some massage oil or lotion handy. Use liberally.

6. Do lots of caressing all over the body before you even begin to sexually stimulate one another.

7. Have fun!

Medical Treatment

If you obtained a score under 17, you may be suffering from physical aspects of impotence. A visit with your doctor is definitely in order. First of all, check on the possible effects of any medication your physician may have prescribed and consider alternative drugs or treatments. That, in itself, may alleviate the problem.

Have a complete physical, keeping a special lookout for diabetes, atherosclerosis or neurological diseases, such as Parkinson's or epilepsy. Be sure, as well, that your doctor checks you out for hormonal abnormalities, especially testosterone.

The Pros and Cons of Testosterone Therapy

Living ten years longer presents a challenge to men whose testosterone levels decrease somewhat as the years go by, resulting in a slightly diminishing sex drive. Men in their 60s and older tend to take longer to get an erection and to achieve orgasm, but there's more to lovemaking than a fast erection and quick ejaculation. Less driven by an urgent sex drive, older men can be exquisite lovers. They can now pay more attention to their lover's needs and take the time to satisfy them. Most women appreciate this, and prefer the more experienced lover to a younger, but more self-centered, stud.

Living ten years longer offers new challenges to intimacy in a loving relationship. We're quite familiar with the prospect of menopause in the midlife woman, but in the past few years, there's been a growing awareness of the question of male menopause. The main concern is the decreasing levels of testosterone, resulting in lowered sex drive.

Every problem has a solution, and so medical technology came up with the testosterone patch. If smokers could get nicotine through their skin by using a transdermal patch, why couldn't a similar technology deliver testosterone?

One company in Palo Alto came up with such a patch and has submitted it to the FDA for approval. This patch must be worn on the scrotum, from which the removal of the patch may not be so pleasant. A rival company in Salt Lake City has tested a similar patch that can be worn anywhere on the body. Much better!

But who benefits most from such a patch? Well, there's no clear answer to that. Only about 10 percent of men between the ages of 20 and 40 suffer from testosterone deficiency. After age 40, it climbs steadily to 15 percent of men and after age 65, it climbs to 20 percent of all men.

Whether testosterone is the main culprit or not is uncertain, but we do know that as we age our sexual desire begins to decline. Occasional impotency affects about 20 percent of all men by age 55, about 30 percent by age 65, and over 50 percent by age 75.

Testosterone, whether by patch or by injection, is not the best solution for declining sexuality. One unfortunate side effect of such hormone therapy is the finding that supplemental testosterone can encourage the problem of benign prostate enlargement and possible prostate cancer as well.

Benign prostate enlargement is simply the slight tendency of the normal prostate gland to grow larger with age. Many men over 50 and a majority of those over 75 will suffer from this. By itself this is no great cause for concern, unless it interferes with normal urination.

The greater concern is the occasional prostate cancer which occasionally accompanies prostate enlargement. In any case, supplemental testosterone only encouragea this dangerous possibility. Some researchers even believe that raising the testosterone level may actually trigger the development of prostate enlargement or cancer.

Keep Your Sex Organs Young and Strong Through Technology

We've spent a good deal of time in this chapter dealing with the many factors of sex, love, and relationships as well as the problems of impotence as they relate to the maturation process of a man's life. It might be appropriate to look at how to fine-tune the sexuality of ten more years in order to keep it as intense and active as we'd like. There's a technology available to us that can compensate for whatever decreases there may be in sex drive as we mature. During these special extra years—the 70s, 80s and even 90s—men's erections may become less spontaneous, less rigid, with more time elapsing between erections. Although this allows for more intimate foreplay between the lovers, allowing for more tenderness and emotional closeness, some may choose to enhance their sexual prowess with modern medical technology. Although medical proof does not exist claiming the benefits of rhinoceros tusk and ginseng root, there is one substance that has proven effective as an aphrodisiac of sorts for men. The African substance, *yohimbine*, proved successful as a sexual stimulant with animals and prodded American researchers to experiment with a related compound called *papaverine*. This substance, when injected directly into the penis shaft, created long-lasting erections for half the men tested.

Suction Pumps

For those men who seek more dependable assistance, there are erection-aid devices such as suction pumps, and penile implants. The suction pump is a hand-operated device that fits over the penis. Suction draws blood into the penis, resulting in an otherwise natural erection. A study of this device showed that 91 percent of the men attempting to use it found it enabled them to have successful intercourse after a brief instruction session at their doctor's office.

Semirigid Implants

Surgical implants offer another option for assured sexuality in those ten special years. Two versions are available. In the simpler of the two, a semi-rigid device is implanted in the penis surgically. At least three such models have proven safe and effective. The disadvantage of such surgery is that it leaves the man with a constant semi-erection.

Inflatable Implants

A more naturally performing sexuality is achieved by the somewhat more complex, multicomponent inflatable penile prosthesis. Hollow cylinders, implanted in the penis, are connected to a reservoir containing a fluid and operated by a small, round pump, conveniently located in the scrotum. Available since 1973, these sexual aids are becoming more and more refined. Some of the newer models are getting rave reviews from their users. Of 332 men using one of them, 83 percent were quite satisfied, and only 16 percent required repeat surgery for minor repairs. A two-year follow-up of 80 men using another model revealed good overall satisfaction and no development of mechanical problems.

Powerful Feelings of Social Confidence

But the quality of sex in those special years should not be defined in the light of reliance on medical science alone. Sex can be great for many even during this period without such assistance. It is there for those who need or want it. But for most, sex is just as sweet in its natural state during this period. The most important qualities for an active sex life, at any age, are a powerful feeling of adequacy and self-worth, along with a strong sense of social involvement. Any man with a general sense of confidence about his standing within his social group is likely also to be successful as a sexual being. So long as we stay active and maintain a strong sense of self-efficacy, we can anticipate staying sexually active and satisfied.

PROLONG YOUR LIFE WITH CANCER SCREENING

Testicular cancer is the most common type of cancer in white men aged 20 to 34. Yet very few men have heard about self-examination for testicular cancer. This type of cancer can spread easily to other organs, causing rapid death. But 90 percent of these cases can be cured by surgery. So the testicular self-exam (TSE) is very important. Here's how to do it.

This is best done during or after a warm shower, when the scrotum (the sac holding the testicles) is loose and relaxed.

Gently roll each testicle between the thumbs and fingers, checking for lumps, swelling, or other unusual features. A normal testicle feels smooth, egg-shaped, and rather firm. One testicle may be larger than the other—that's normal.

First, you'll feel the epididymis. That's the string-like structure on the top and back of each testicle that stores and transports sperm. Then feel around for any small, hard, pea-sized lumps. These are the lumps to worry about, even if they're painless. Any lump, unusual tenderness, enlargement of the scrotum, pain, or feeling of heaviness should be reported to your doctor.

When testicular cancer is suspected, the usual way to confirm the diagnosis is with surgery, to remove the entire affected testicle. The remaining testicle can still supply sufficient sperm and hormones so that fertility and sexual function are not at all impaired.

WHAT TO DO ABOUT PROSTATE CONDITIONS

Many men have heard of the prostate gland in recent years because of public health efforts to inform the public about cancer threats, but not all understand exactly what it is and what its function is.

First of all, the prostate is *not* a sex organ in itself, but it does play a significant role in sexual reproduction. Its main function is to produce the seminal fluid that supports the sperm to be ejaculated through the penis. It makes about 90 percent of the milky semen in which the sperm travel.

In the adult male, the prostate is about the size and shape of a large walnut and surrounds the urethra, the tube that carries urine from the bladder to the penis. It lies just before the sphincter muscle that men can use to voluntarily control the flow of urine. So when you contract that muscle, you're close to the prostate gland. It also lies just below the bladder and next to the inner wall of the rectum. The prostate consists of 5 lobes, most of which can be felt by a physician when he inserts his index finger into the rectum. This is the most common medical examination for the health of this gland.

Symptoms

By the time you're 60 years of age, chances are you'll be having some symptom of prostatic disorder. But it may occur much earlier as well. The digital rectal exam (which should be an annual even after age 40) will probably provide the first indication of abnormality, unless infection or overgrowth create symptoms before that. Such symptoms will occur in one of three ways:

1. Urgent need to urinate or unusual frequency

2. Discomfort or pain during urination

3. Pain in the pelvic area

Upon hearing such complaints, your doctor will most likely update your medical history, do a rectal exam, and do a urinalysis. In some cases, he may decide to do a cystoscopy—view the urethra and bladder areas through a special viewing instrument that goes through the penis. But, fortunately, this is rather rare.

Here are some of the conditions he might end up diagnosing:

1. *Bacterial infection, or common prostatitis.* This occurs in younger men as well as older ones. Usually it's a spread of infection from the bladder or urethra. Symptoms can include lower-abdominal pain and fever.

2. *Nonbacterial prostatitis.* This congestion occurs when too much fluid accumulates in the gland. This is commonly believed to be due to stress factors. Some doctors think that this may also be caused by too much or too little sex. It's most likely the abrupt change that is the cause—not too much or too little by itself.

3. *Nonspecific urethritis* (NSU). This is not actually an inflammation of the prostate itself but rather of the part of the urethra passing through it. This is usually caused by chlamydia, the most common sexually-transmitted disease.

4. *Benign prostatic hyperplasia* (BPH). This is more commonly referred to as noncancerous enlargement of the prostate, which is fairly normal in men as they age, particularly after age 50. This increase in size is normally as much as 50 percent over the size it was in his 20s and 30s. Some of this growth is inward and a problem occurs when it begins to choke off the urethra through which the urine flows, causing difficulty in urination or urinary frequency (having to get up during the night, and so on.)

By age 50, half the men have BPH and by age 70, 75 percent have it. By age 80, it's almost a foregone conclusion. In the U.S., about 10 million men over age 50 report problems due to BPH. It's responsible for 1.7 million doctor visits a year and some 400,000 operations.

5. *Prostate cancer.* This is a very slow-growing cancer that is unusually common, especially as men get older. One third of men over age 50 have microscopic evidence of it—but it is usually not fatal. Seventy percent of men over 80 have it, yet they die of other causes, not prostate cancer. In other words, they outlive the cancer and die of another ailment or natural occurence.

The actual symptoms of the above conditions are different for the first three from the last two. For infection of the prostate, men will typically find the opening of the penis seeming to be "glued" shut upon wakening in the morning. When forced open manually, a drop or two of clear liquid can be seen. At the end of the day, they may find a brownish or yellowish stain in their underwear, a sign of infection. They may also feel a sense of itching or discomfort within the urethra of the penis, as well as discomfort when urinating.

Overgrowth of the prostate (BPH) and related cancer possibilities will be experienced as the difficulty or hesitancy in urinating as well as urinary frequency, as previously mentioned.

One way to distinguish serious infection of the prostate from NSU or nonbacterial inflammation is by the high fever (as high as 102 degrees or even higher) and flu-like aches and pains as well as abdominal and lower-back pain. You'll definitely want to see your doctor at this point.

Prevention for Enlarged Prostate

Since Asian men seem to suffer from BPH only after they've migrated to the West, it's believed that a low-cholesterol, low-fat diet is the way to go.

In addition to that, zinc supplements of 50 mg./day may help. Or you can get the zinc in such foods as chicken, peas, lentils, wheat germ, and bran.

Homeopaths recommend cold-pressed linseed oil or a pollen preparation called *cernitin*.

Because pumpkin seeds were an important part of the diet among Transylvanians where BPH was almost nonexistent, some doctors believe this food may impart good prostatic health. Pumpkin seeds, of course, happen to be high in zinc.

Vitamins considered essential for a healthy prostate gland are, in daily dosage:

1. Vitamin A, from 5,000 to 20,000 International Units (IU)

2. Vitamin C, from 200 to 500 mg.

3. Vitamin D, 400 IU

4. Vitamin E, 30 to 100 IU

In addition, essential fatty acid capsules up to 1,200 mg./day, one or two tablespoons of lecithin and 3 pollen tablets a day are recommended for a healthy prostate gland.

Solutions for Enlarged Prostate

Once you've been diagnosed with BPH, there are seven possibilities to be considered:

1. *Self-treatment.* This involves getting your supply of zinc and other supplements as I've just mentioned, along with a homeopathic treatment consisting of a combination of three amino acids: *alanine, glutamate,* and *glycine,* taking several grams of this a day. If you want to go all out in this self-treatment, you might also include lecithin and calcium and magnesium tablets.

2. *Medication.* There are 3 categories of medication that you can explore with your doctor.

   a. The first group is made up of antihypertensive drugs, the same drugs that are used to combat high blood pressure. Although still in the research stages, these drugs can relax the muscle tissue in the prostate, easing the pressure on the urethra.

   b. The second group works by affecting the metabolism of testosterone. In this group is the only drug specifically approved by the FDA to treat BPH. It's *finasteride,* better known as *Proscar,* because of the direct marketing to the consumer by its manufacturer, Merck.

   Proscar is particularly effective in shrinking enlarged prostates and keeping them shrunk. But unfortunately it only helps half the men who take it. Also, it's expensive. At 5 mg./day, the cost adds up to about $650 a year. And for those for whom it works, it must be taken for life. When treatment is stopped, symptoms return within two weeks.

   c. A third category under investigation is known as *aromatase inhibitors,* which block the action of converting testosterone into a form of estrogen that may contribute to BPH. This category is only in the early stages of research at this time.

What does the future hold? Merck is working hard on a more potent "son of Proscar" which would be even more effective. I imagine a combination of the three categories of drugs I've just described would be the ideal medical solution to this very common problem.

3. *Surgery*. A prostatectomy involves removing the new tissue that is a result of BPH both at the outer capsule as well as the part of the urethra surrounded by the enlarged prostate. Healing allows for a new lining for the passageway growing naturally from the bladder end of the urethra.

Most surgery nowadays avoids cutting through the abdomen and instead goes through the urethra and cuts the inner-most core of the prostate. This has been compared to a "Roto-rooter" job. The special instrument goes through the penis to the middle of the prostate where a tubular knife blade cuts away the engorging tissue while electric currents seal off any bleeding vessels.

Another, less complicated procedure involves getting to the same area and merely cutting two deep incisions from the bladder neck through the prostate, thus widening the urinary passage.

Whether or not to have surgery is purely an option dictated by the discomfort of BPH. If a man is not too upset by the symptoms of BPH he can wait as long as he wishes to have surgery unless, of course, there are other factors to consider.

4. *Microwave probe*. In this procedure, a microwave probe called a *prostatron*, is passed through the urethra, destroying the surrounding tissue by heating it to 113 degrees Fahrenheit. This damaged tissue is then absorbed by the body. Using a cooling system to keep the urethra from being damaged, the treatment is effective at its first and only administration, doing away with the need to come back to the doctor for any additional treatments that may have been necessary before the cooling system was employed. This new treatment is still under investigation by the FDA and looks very promising.

5. TULIP (*Transurethral Ultrasound-guided Laser-Induced Prostatectomy*). As in the microwave technique, a probe is inserted through the penis with an ultrasound probe and laser. The ultrasound image helps the doctor find the proper location where the laser beam heats the prostate tissue. This burned tissue is slowly absorbed by the body, as in the microwave technique.

6. *Balloon dilation.* Again, as in the techniques just described, a probe enters through the urethra, this time with a balloon attached to the tip. When the urethra surrounded by the prostate is reached, the balloon is inflated to about 1 inch for about 10 to 15 minutes.

Although this relatively simple treatment is already approved by the FDA, it appears to be successful for only a few months to 2 years. Consequently, this technique is typically used as a short-term option when more radical surgery must be delayed or as a mild treatment for those with moderate symptoms.

7. A *reinforced "tunnel."* In this treatment, a spring-like cylinder called a *stent* is inserted through the urethra. Its tubular metal mesh anchors itself in the afflicted area once it's inserted. This is the simplest technique of all, yet highly effective, and requires the least amount of hospitalization. It also provides a happy alternative to older men who are too affected by heart or lung disease to undergo surgery.

Detecting Cancer of the Prostate

1. The most common diagnostic technique is the infamous digital rectal exam. The test is not at all difficult; just relax and trust your doctor. The rest is easy. Within a few seconds you're relieved of any discomfort whatsoever, because the test itself is that brief. And, best of all, that's it for another year.

   You also enjoy the assurance that you've done your part in detection against a cancer that is present, at least in microscopic form, with a probability of occurrence at 50 percent in all men over 50. It is the most common serious cancer affecting men. It develops slowly and is most curable when detected early. So a few seconds of slight discomfort every year is worth it, don't you think? Early detection of small cancers and subsequent surgery will add years to your life.

   Once a year, after age 40, make sure you have a digital rectal exam by your doctor. He or she will be able to feel if there are any tumors in the prostate and detect any cancer in its earliest stages.

2. Even more sensitive and certainly less uncomfortable is the popular *Prostate-Specific Antigen test.* Prostate-Specific Antigen

(PSA) is a normal secretion of the prostate, but increases significantly even in the early stages of cancer growth. The test is far from perfect, giving false results—both positive and negative—one third to one half of the time. But since prostate cancers grow slowly and the PSA test can be taken on a regular basis over time, the test will hopefully be a help to you. This test should be an annual "must" for you if you have a family history of prostate cancer, if you're an African-American over age 50, or if you're of any race over age 65.

Preventing Cancer of the Prostate

In the U.S., at least 38,000 men will die of prostate cancer each year. There is at least one way you can help avoid being part of this statistic.

Research on nearly 48,000 men over 4 years has revealed that although there is no correlation between diet and "latent" prostate cancer—small tumors that can lie dormant for decades—there is a strong relationship between the consumption of saturated fat, particularly from red meat, and the incidence of advanced cancers. The researchers suspect these are the carcinogens that form when meat is cooked.

Cross-cultural research indicates that advanced prostate cancers are most common where the diet has the highest proportion of fat. So the best preventive measure against the problems of prostate cancer is to avoid eating meat.

Solution for Prostate Cancer

If the cancer is diagnosed as being restricted to only one area and you're over 70, your doctor may decide to follow you closely without any surgery or other treatment. If you're younger or if the cancer is not contained to one area, then surgery and/or radiation or chemotherapy may be prescribed.

Cancer of the prostate is among the most curable. Seventy-one percent survive for more than five years after being diagnosed with this cancer.

SIX STEPS IN KEEPING YOUR PROSTATE YOUNG AND STRONG

Now that you know all the details of what could go wrong with your prostate, how to detect it, prevent it, and the possible solutions, here is a six-step summary of what to do on a day-to-day basis.

1. Know Your Options

Much more common than prostate cancer is the benign, non-cancerous enlargement of the prostate that's so very common among over-50 males. As this process develops, it eventually causes resistance to urination and therefore more frequent trips to the bathroom at night as well as other discomforts. Surgery (through the urethra) is the traditional treatment. Some attempt microwave treatment, a single, 90-minute application, which has proved to reduce frequency of bathroom visits from 12 to 7 in a 24-hour period.

2. See Your Doctor

In addition, there are two medications that help ease the problem. One relaxes the prostate muscle, reducing the pressure on the urethra; and the other helps to shrink the gland itself. The downside is that it'll take six months or so to see if they will work for you. They don't work for everyone.

3. Less Fat and Meat

In a nutshell, sharply decrease your intake of fat, and avoid red meat, and salt-cured or smoked luncheon meats. Include more high-fiber cereals, as well as fruits and vegetables, especially such cruciferous vegetables as brussels sprouts, cabbage, broccoli, and cauliflower, which contain natural factors to help the body detoxify carcinogens. Plus, don't overlook your vitamin and mineral supplements. Vitamins A, B_6, C, and E as well as the minerals calcium and selenium play particularly important roles.

4. Drink Less in the Evening

Although prostate enlargement is common in over-50 males, only about one man in five will have symptoms severe enough to require any medical treatment. In the meantime, the best approach to mild versions of the problem is to avoid long intervals between urination and, in order to get a good night's sleep, to limit fluid intake in the evening.

5. Jog or Walk

Research has shown that exercise helps deter cancer of the prostate. According to a Harvard University study of over 17,000 alumni, since testosterone levels are thought to be related to the development of prostate cancer, the exercise lowers testosterone levels and therefore the risk of prostate cancer. But you need to be doing about 8 hours of jogging a week or walking 40 miles a week for this preventive measure. That's about 4 to 6 miles of jogging a day. If jogging is your exercise of choice, then this is just added incentive.

6. Maintain Your Healthy Lifestyle

As I mentioned, only one in five who have mild symptoms of prostate enlargement will get worse, three in five will remain the same, and one in five will actually improve. So the news is not all bad. In the meantime, as preventive measures against prostate cancer, keep up with your fitness program and follow the guidelines for proper nutrition as suggested in the chapters on those topics.

— SIDEBAR I —

NONTRADITIONAL ALTERNATIVE TO TREATMENT OF BPH

The traditional treatment for overgrowth of the prostate (BPH) is the drug *Proscar,* which works by affecting the metabolism of testosterone.

Yet, according to the *Physicians' Desk Reference,* the doctor's "Bible" on drugs, a comparison with the natural herb, *saw palmetto (Serenoa repens),* indicates that the natural herb is 38 percent more effective in enhancing the rate of urine flow after only three months of treatment. As a matter of fact, even though

Proscar is effective in only half the men treated even after a year, saw palmetto is effective with 90 percent of men, usually within a four- to six-week period.

Saw palmetto has been used for centuries as a folk medicine not only to treat the prostate, but also as an aphrodisiac and sex rejuvenator. Saw palmetto, at a dosage of 320 mg./day, has been clinically researched in over ten studies, and the results of these studies all concur that significant improvement can be obtained in terms of enhanced urine flow.

The Food and Drug Administration has approved Proscar but chose to reject saw palmetto as a treatment for BPH despite the natural herb's clear scientifically proven superiority to Proscar, despite its greater proven safety in terms of side effects, and despite its less expensive cost.

If you're wondering why, you might want to educate yourself about the larger manufacturers lobbying governmental agencies. In the meantime, if you want to try saw palmetto for yourself, try a dosage of 160 mg. twice daily. It can be obtained at most health-food stores as a supplement.

THE MIDLIFE YEARS: GETTING YOUR SECOND WIND

Sometime during a man's forties or fifties, a midlife crisis, characterized by self-doubt, depressive thinking, and concerns about aging can be precipitated by a serious personal illness, the death of a parent or close friend, a career failure or a disruption of his marriage. Male menopause—with sexual concern as a main focus—may occur a few years later or actually coincide with the main midlife crisis in a man's life. In other words, male menopause is a special type of midlife crisis. In this first section, we focus on the more general category of midlife crisis.

MIDLIFE CRISIS: UNDERSTANDING THE CAUSES

Sometime in their mid-forties, both Charles Dickens and Paul Gauguin left their wives and families for greener pastures. Dickens took up with a 16-year-old and Gauguin left his staid bank career and headed for the South Seas where he could paint to his heart's content. What causes such abrupt shifts in a man's life? Here are seven factors.

1. Does Life Begin or End at 40?

Although we're told it begins at 40, it doesn't seem that way to many turning that age. Letting go of the 30s and entering the 40s seems like a monumental shift for many men. They grieve for the lost youth that is so glamorized and revered in our culture.

2. "September Song"

Reaching the halfway point of life (assuming 80 years of life), these men now look ahead to see what awaits them and what they see off in the horizon of their lifespan is a gradual deterioration—more physical vulnerability, a withering of their physical prowess, and ulti-mately, the eternal nothingness of death. Such fears of decline into old age may appear silly to the onlooker, but for such men struck hard by midlife crises, there's nothing ahead to look forward to but triviality, meaninglessness, stagnation, and hopelessness.

3. Midlife Confusion

As the midlife shift takes place, it's felt abruptly and there's no man-ual or set of guidelines on how to adjust older value systems to deal with the new parameters of life. Men feel thrown from youth to matu-rity overnight with no road map to guide them. They feel as confused and vulnerable as they were on their first day of school.

4. Changing Relationships

One of the causes of the crisis may be a new-found love, either with someone they've found for themselves or someone their *spouses* have found. Or it may be children leaving home for college or a career opportunity. The "empty nest" syndrome can spark a midlife crisis just as easily as a faltering marriage.

5. Psychological Milestones

Carl Jung understood the shift into maturity better than any other psychotherapist, as indicated in his description of the process he called *individuation*, in which a man's personality shifts from manliness to his more feminine side. All the softer characteristics are now released to the surface, allowing for expression of a gentleness and sensitivity covered until now by a macho mask.

Erik Erikson covered the eight stages of a person's development and characterized the midlife crisis as a battle between *generativity* (extending oneself to family, society, and future generations) on the one hand, and *self-absorption* (concern with only material possessions and physical well-being) on the other. Caught between a rock and a hard place, psychologically speaking, men in midlife crisis may be like the famous photo of the raccoon holding on to the dock with its left legs and the boat drifting away with its right legs. It can't let go and it can't hold on—a crisis indeed!

6. Midlife Ceiling

Just as the women's movement has coined the term "glass ceiling," referring to the level beyond which women will not be promoted, regardless of their talent and drive, so there is a "midlife ceiling," beyond which those men who are no longer "young" will no longer be promoted. This ceiling may not be as clear-cut as the glass ceiling, but it exists nonetheless, and is as much an insult to men's personal pride as the glass ceiling is to a woman's serve of pride.

7. Ultimate Questions

Finally, any or all these shocks to the psyche of the midlife male confront him with the ultimate questions of his life to date. What have I accomplished in my life so far? Where am I headed and is it the right direction for me? What is my life all about, anyway? If he gets depressed enough, he may even ask himself: Is the struggle worth it after all?

Frank was a 43-year-old architect who was going through as severe a midlife crisis as I'd ever seen in my practice. He'd left his devoted wife of 20 years and was living with his mistress, though he still had a strong emotional connection to his wife. He was so wracked with guilt and indecision that he couldn't even attend to his profession in any effective way. He was holding on to a romantic image of his younger life by "shacking up" with his mistress, but wasn't willing to let go of the life-long relationship he had with his wife.

His sexual response to his wife had dimmed, but his much younger mistress turned him on without fail. At the same time, Frank realized that building a new life with his mistress just wouldn't fill the bill. His friends would never accept this arrangement and he wasn't willing to give up his network of friends either.

Frank was able to share his feelings so much more openly with his mistress who loved him devotedly and without many demands. His wife, on the other hand, was by now filled with hurt and bitterness for obvious reasons. She didn't want to give up the marriage but had little control over her husband's doings.

To make things worse, Frank's lack of attention to his profession was causing a financial bind that impinged on all three participants in this midlife triangle. Things were getting increasingly desperate as his visits to my office increased in frequency. Frank was becoming increasingly depressed and debilitated.

Frank's midlife crisis finally came to a happy resolution. Our discussions focused on the importance of his family life and the impact his leaving home had on his children. Frank sold his share of the business to his partner and took a job in sales—a job with less responsibility and more freedom to enjoy his hobby of sculpting, an expression he'd been denying himself.

Frank felt this crisis had been a learning experience for him. He decided to share what he'd learned in a relationship class that he led at church. He was able to enjoy this forum for sharing with others the deeper appreciation he now felt for commitment and honest communication. Frank had his "new" relationship of openness and honesty not only with his wife but also with his children, who could now really enjoy their "new" father.

Frank began to exercise regularly and eat more wisely than he had before. He even invited his son to work out with him, nurturing this "new" relationship. He entered his sculpture into a contest and won a prize for his innovative and original style. He finally felt affirmed as a husband, father, provider, and artist. Frank was as happy as I'd ever seen him.

Can you relate to any part of this story? More than you care to admit, perhaps? If so, then guess what!

Yes, you're in midlife crisis. It's later than you think. It's farther than you'd like down the road of your life. So this is the time to do what you'll be proud of when your headstone is made public. If you're not headed in that direction, then make use of your moral compass and turn accordingly. What is your life all about, indeed! It's about you, your dreams, your potential, your uniqueness.

OVERCOMING YOUR MIDLIFE CRISIS

As you can see, a midlife crisis can take a number of shapes, male menopause being just one of them. Overcoming the cycle of depressive, self-critical thinking is not easy. That's exactly why such radical decisions as choosing a younger woman or abandoning a career for "artistic" pursuits are such easy outs. The real challenge is to come to grips with the reality of your life situation, to foster a solution that works out for the best in the long run and that does not devastate those who love you and depend on you.

1. Life Really Does Begin at 40

According to Confucius, at age 40 we can finally transcend our perplexities. The mysteries of life can be viewed somewhat more clearly. We can separate the important from the trivial. Our priorities can be held with greater conviction. We really do know, finally, what it's all about—at least much more than we did previously. According to the sacred Talmud, reaching 40 is the transition from focusing on physical strength to mental strength, and understanding the world around us.

2. "And These Few Precious Days. . . ."

Yes, "September Song" laments the passage of time as "the days dwindle down to a precious few," but more important are the words, "One hasn't got time for the waiting game." As you enter midlife, don't waste time sitting around waiting for opportunity to knock, or to be recognized for your hidden worth. Now you can give yourself permission to move out and forge ahead with what's really important to you. To quote the Talmud again:

> "If you are not for yourself, then who will be?
> If you are for yourself alone, then who are you?
> And if not now, while you are young, then when?"

I'll paraphrase: If not now, when overcoming your midlife crisis, then when?

3. Developing into a New, Confident Being

According to Solon, throughout the 40s and into the 50s is the time when "the tongue and the mind. . . together are now at their best." This is the time to begin speaking your mind, whether as a teacher, counselor, or leader. As a successful public speaker myself, I've often wondered why most of the successful speakers are mature individuals in their 40s and more often in their 50s and 60s. Of course, it takes time to build success. But beyond that, I've come to realize that it takes a certain amount of having lived life before one is really ready to speak with confidence from the platform. Yes, life begins at 40, in the sense that you're now ready to be fully recognized for your convictions. Your ability to teach, counsel, and support others through your wisdom is not an obligation. It's a calling—a very meaningful one and highly enjoyable when done well.

4. New Relationships

A new-found love does not usually have the lasting power of your ongoing one. Sure, there's the high drama of novelty and intrigue and that should be fun for a few weeks or months, but typically the superficial aspects of a relationship based on sexual passion soon wear thin. And unless your ongoing relationship endures, you may be a very lonely man. The "new" woman in your life may be none other than the one who's always been with you, the "newness" having more to do with a new respect for her and openness to communication and allowing the mutual vulnerabilities of a life shared together to occur. Even your children can become new friends as you open up to one another as real human beings, transcending your conventional roles as parents and children.

5. Passing Through the Psychological Milestones

As you confront the passage of what Jung referred to as individuation, you can enjoy letting go of your male armor, the need always to appear strong and invincible. You can let the emotions you've been suppressing come to full expression—laughter, tears, joy, and sadness. You can explore those creative urges that were always pushed aside because of "important" matters. Let the artist, the musician in you come out of hiding. It's in there, in every one of you.

As for Erikson's crisis between self-absorption and generativity, let go of the former and embrace the latter. Sure, it's important to stay healthy and youthful, to follow the guidelines I've suggested in this book so far. But, beyond that, don't dwell on your physical appearance. Stay trim, eat smart, groom yourself nicely, and then move on to your family, share your hard-earned wisdom with the younger generation, enjoy your capacity for leadership in your community, profession, or even to promote the social values you hold dear in a political setting. Reach out to the world and be embraced by it in turn.

6. Midlife Boost

Tired of 10-hour work days for the past decade or two? Like Charlie Chaplin in *Modern Days*, tightening an endless steam of nuts and bolts at breakneck pace got you down? Sick of being held back by the midlife ceiling while all those young studs around you are promoted over your head? Then brighten up! Here's your chance to turn it all around in your favor.

By the time you hit midlife, you've got a pretty good idea of what you do better than anyone else. You also happen to enjoy it because you're a natural at it. However, you have to deal with one harsh reality: If you're going to choose your life path instead of having it chosen for you, chances are you'll have to take a substantial cut in pay—at least in the short run.

So you must decide: Keep selling your soul to the devil, for a price (your current salary), or become the captain of your fate (financially bloodied but unbowed). You can give up being a school teacher in Decatur and make no money for a few years while you get your Ph.D. or M.D. James Workhard, Ph.D., or James Workhard, M.D.— which sounds better to you? It's there for the asking (and a few years of sacrifice!). The money will then come, though there's absolutely no correlation between income and happiness according to many informal interviews over the years.

"But," you interject with conviction, "what about my kids? I can't let them down. How will I support their lifestyle, their schooling? I can't drag them into poverty with me!" Well, imagine your parents in a similar dilemma. Which would you have them choose? Would you have them sacrifice their dreams for your sake or would you support them in this cause and hang together as a loving family through thick and thin (wallet)?

I realize this is an unnerving suggestion. But this whole exercise of considering such a radical move is to get you out of your midlife slump. At this point, you're in a better position to do a fair evaluation of your current situation as compared to your fantasy. The juices of ambition are flowing and you're excited about the possibilities. So now is the time to make that proverbial list of all the pros and cons of both possibilities. Only you can add up the points for either side—financial points, emotional points, parental responsibility points, and so on—and let your gut break the tie, if it gets that close. Your gut is much better at this than your brain.

Whatever your decision, the midlife ceiling has been shattered. Your fate is back in your hands.

7. Ultimate Answers

So what have you accomplished in your life so far? If not much, in your estimation, then this is the time to change things. Imagine yourself at your own funeral and looking down at your own headstone. What would you want engraved on it?

UNDERSTANDING MALE MENOPAUSE

Humility—a term not often used by virile-looking men in the prime of life. Yet it is the most accurate description of how men feel when, in their 50s, they first experience the failure of their penis. Even with an attractive, willing, loving woman at their bedside, the penis fails to respond. They can feel abject failure, disappointment, panic about this midlife crisis, but beyond all that, an underlying sense of humility. "Absence of pride or self-assertion," according to Webster's definition of humility, says it just as well.

A Common Occurrence

Successful, healthy men in the throes of midlife success all have this in common: their sexual drive is found to be diminishing. No longer as easily aroused as they were a mere 5 or 10 years ago, their erections neither as frequent nor always as rock-hard as they used to be, their ejaculations sometimes a mere sputtering compared to the cannon-like blasts of their youth, they are forced to concede to a shift in sex drive and energy that makes them less competitive in the sexual arena, if competitive is indeed what they choose to be.

A Lonely Crisis

With whom can they talk about this? With their wives, whose own menopausal crises create their own problems? With their mistresses, whom they will surely lose if they openly admit to such sexual frailty? With their buddies, who are still cracking sophomoric jokes about sexual machismo? With their family doctors, who may have contributed to the problem by prescribing some tranquilizer or blood pressure medicine? With their ministers, who are likely to sweep the problem under the rug, and suggest marriage encounter? Male menopause is a lonely crisis!

Ignoring It Won't Make It Go Away

Many wonder about the evidence for such a catch-all term as *male menopause*. There is hardly any mention of it in the medical literature. There are only a mere handful of books on the topic, a few published in the 1970s and very few since then. The Europeans seem more comfortable with the concept than we Americans. In England, they call it *viropause*. In Europe, it's referred to as *andropause*. In the United States, we tend to ignore it—as in, maybe it'll go away.

But it's all too prevalent, too troublesome a challenge to ignore. And if we try overlooking it or sweeping it under the rug in one fashion or another, it can lead to a form of midlife crisis. So rather than attempt to ignore it, let's tackle it head on, to use a good old macho football term.

From the time the hormone testosterone begins to flush through a boy's body at puberty until he reaches 40, normal problems of sexual dysfunction can fit into a thimble, compared to the bushels needed to take up the problems encountered in the 20 years following.

The *Age-40-Paradox* occurs just at the height of sexual mastery and confidence. The youthful/mature male may begin to notice some undeniable changes in his sexuality. Although he's learned to take pride in the self-control he's mastered over his sexual response, he may soon realize that this change is in one direction only—slower— and less and less under his own control.

Particularly for those reaching 40 who smoke, drink alcohol regularly, or overeat without exercising, the change is more noticeable. Regular smoking damages the blood vessels leading to the penis, resulting in more difficulty in attaining erections. Years of chronic alcoholism damage the nerves inside the penis, making it less sensitive to stimulation. High blood cholesterol levels seem related to a higher incidence of impotency. So by age 40, poor health habits begin to catch up with him.

At what I call *Age-50-Crisis*, there is a shift downward in the level of testosterone for about one third of men. This downward shift is very complex. Although only one man in ten at this juncture will suffer a substantial drop in overall level, about one in five will suffer a precipitous drop in what's referred to as free or available testosterone—that component taking part in sexual arousal. One result of this is that such men may now need physical stimulation in addition to the visual stimulation which sufficed in younger years. A greater degree of stimulation overall is required for sexual arousal.

By Age-50-Crisis, such factors as smoking and chronic alcoholism have an even stronger impact. Sex drive is noticeably reduced and it may take somewhat longer than usual to become aroused sexually. Ejaculations tend to be less forceful and the volume of emitted semen is reduced. Because sexual arousal does not come that easily, many at this age are tempted to increase the intensity of stimulation under their control. They may rely more and more on pornography or new erotically interesting—often younger—partners. They may find themselves more often in a position of paying for sexual arousal, rather than earning it by dint of their charm or attractiveness as they had in younger years.

An emotional transformation begins here; feelings of sexual vulnerability begin to prevail. Since this is the age most men are susceptible to male menopause, they may become temporarily impotent as they suffer the full force of this malady. The working through of this sexual crisis involves a thorough exploration of life values, involving career decisions, open communication with their mates, and a decision to take charge of health factors in their lives.

Assuming they work through this crisis with family support and professional guidance in relatively short order, a satisfactory adjustment can be made, with anticipation of a more meaningful sexuality than they experienced premenopause.

What Is Male Menopause?

First of all, let's be precise about what it is we're discussing. Male menopause is a physical condition with emotional consequences. The physical condition is the natural midlife aging process with particular focus on the decreasing sexual drive inherent in that process. At its worst, it can result in occasional to chronic impotence with accompanying depression and lowered self-esteem. It usually occurs during the 50s, but can start as early as the late 30s or as late as the 60s.

The Age

Although I've focused on the sexual factor in explaining the onset of male menopause, it is not always so. In many cases, decreasing sex drive is not a factor. Instead, the onset may be precipitated by career or financial crises, or other major setbacks. In such cases, decrease in sex drive may be the result, rather than the cause, of male menopause. A physical change is still central to the process, but this may be a decrease in energy or the body's ability to cope with major stresses that lead to emotional consequences. In my interviews with men, it seems as if 52 is the most likely age at which this awareness of midlife transition takes place. Certainly, the early 50s is the most likely period for male menopause to be first acknowledged.

The Causes

The reason I've focused on decrease in sexuality as a precipitating factor is because that particular crisis is so important to the male ego that it's the proverbial two-by-four upside-the-head that most easily grabs a man's attention. Precipitating factors, other than a decrease in sex drive, can be decreases in physical energy and capacity as well as crises in relationship, career, or finances—whatever it takes to grab a man's attention long enough to make him sit up and take notice that he's no longer the young stud he's spent his life becoming. He's finally forced to take notice that his body is maturing and now demands thoughtful respect. It's precisely the sudden psychological shift from the category of "youth" to that of "maturity" that creates the shock which precipitates the depression and grieving process at the apparent "sudden" loss of his youthful self-concept.

Discovering the Onset

Society serves notice in an uncannily mundane yet powerful way. In his mail one day, shuffled among bills and advertising circulars, is an undistinguished envelope, the contents of which invite him to join the AARP, for which he's now become eligible. For the uninitiated, those letters stand for the American Association of Retired Persons—an association open to all who have reached the age of 50!

Upon understanding this message for the first time, many a man may drop the envelope and its contents as if he were holding a squirming cockroach. For the first time, he's been targeted as belonging to the "old folks set". Soon, his mail will be complemented by ads that might otherwise be aimed at *old* people—how to keep false teeth from slipping, bargain discounts for bifocals, medications, and so on. That's how society lets him know that some time during the previous night, while calmly asleep, he quietly slipped from youth to—dare I say it—maturity!

So male menopause is not just a matter of decreasing sex drive, although that gets his attention most readily. Rather, it's the sudden, dramatic, psychological shift from one category to another which he's been denying as long as he could in this youth-oriented culture. What forces this shift upon him is an external or physical manifestation such as career crisis or a single incident of sexual failure. The AARP invitation makes it official, as much as if the Federal Government had sent an edict announcing that he could no longer honestly pass himself off as youthful in any personal endeavor, whether in the bedroom or the board room. He's now officially on the other side. It's time to grieve his claim to youth and go through his share of depression, if ever he's going to suffer it in that particular manner. That's the essence of male menopause.

The truth of the sexual matter is that, once male menopause is appropriately confronted, sex drive typically returns to full satisfaction. There's no doubt about the very gradual decrease in sex drive over the decades of a man's life, but there's plenty of drive left to allow for an even more satisfying sex life if he takes a mature (oops, there's that word again) approach to it. Take Jack, for instance.

Jack, a corporate lawyer, had just turned 53. Although he used to have a very sexually compatible relationship with his wife Janet, also a lawyer, he was now virtually impotent with her. His emotional attentions were turning to one of his female colleagues. Although this relationship was not sexual . . . yet.

Janet was devastated. She hadn't done anything wrong. Why was Jack rejecting her? Jack's response was one of confusion. He felt he no longer had anything in common with Janet, that she didn't approve of his friends. Jack would rather spend time at the bar after work where he could chew the fat with his friends, including the female colleague he was favoring with his attention.

When Jack came to see me about his situation, one aspect on which we focused was this first bout with impotence. We discussed the possibility of testosterone injections or patches, but ultimately we decided against this because of our conclusion that his problem was more emotional than physiological.

Further discussion revealed Jack was feeling more depressed than he had in years. He felt his youth was ebbing away. Janet was going through menopause and he found her lack of vaginal lubrication, when he tried making love, an emotional slap in the face. The few times he was able to enter her, Janet seemed to be in pain, though she didn't complain openly. Jack just became too discouraged and stopped initiating; Janet didn't either. And so the distancing began. Jack tried making love once or twice more but quickly lost his erection when confronted by Janet's lack of lubrication. Neither of them talked about it. They no longer touched in bed. Once Janet tried to initiate a conversation, but Jack wasn't in the mood to talk about it. It wasn't brought up again.

Jack's impotence, as time revealed, was more psychological than physiological. Once we had a chance to explore the possibility that he was going through a classic case of male menopause, things came into focus.

Sure, Jack's testosterone levels were decreasing, but there was certainly enough left to keep the sexual fire burning, even though it might require a bit more stroking than when he was younger. We discussed some sexual techniques that he and Janet could use, as well as ways for her to deal with vaginal dryness.

As for Jack accepting his situation, he took a more philosophical view, and we discussed how developing a new perspective for his mission in life was in order. There was a truly sad acceptance of life passing, more rapidly than either of us would like, but as well a realization of how acceptance of his mortality would encourage him to live his life as he truly wished, doing what he really wanted to do, and being more honest with Janet about what he wanted from his marriage.

The passing weeks brought Jack and Janet closer. They decided to move to a new part of town where they'd be happier, to choose their friends on a proactive basis rather than remaining in old, boring relationships that each was accepting as a sacrifice to the other.

Near their new home was a large park where Jack could do some jogging a few times a week. He and Janet took long walks during the evening when weather permitted. And Jack took up badminton on the weekends with some new neighbors. Jack and Janet's relationship was revitalized.

SEVEN COMMON SYMPTOMS OF MALE MENOPAUSE

1. Persistence of Depressive Feelings

A man knows he's suffering from male menopause when there's a depression-like anxiety about his life that he can't pin on any particular thing and that he can't shake off. It's not as severe as a true depression—he's still able to work and enjoy many aspects of life—but there's an obsessive awareness about that letter from AARP. He can't shake the thought that the letter was meant for someone else with a similar-looking name, but he *is* over 50. He realizes, finally, that the computer addressing the label to him had a simple instruction—over age 50. It's no mean-spirited bureaucrat who's out to get him, but simply an undeniable fact: He's reached his 50th birthday.

2. Awareness of Aging

He thinks about the times in the last few years when he was just too tired for sex, the sprained muscle that took longer to heal, that exotic seafood that gave his stomach trouble for the first time, the names of old songs that were on the tip of his tongue yet evaded his memory, his belt becoming tighter: He was now part of the "older" generation.

3. Coincidence with Female Menopause

How does male menopause differ from female menopause? Primarily, female menopause is marked clearly by the irregularity and then complete cessation of menstrual periods. In fact, the term *menopause* comes from the terms meaning a *pause* (really, a cessation) of the *monthly* periodic flow of blood. No such clear-cut event marks the onset of the male menopause. Female menopause is often accompanied by occasional insomnia, night sweats, and hot flashes, but ironically an *increase* in sex drive. This increase is fostered by the sudden emergence from the fears and responsibilities related to possible pregnancy along with an increased self-assurance that normally comes with maturity. Within the body of the menopausal woman, the decrease in female hormones allows the adrenal hormones to play a larger role in driving up the libido or sex drive. In many women, even the clitoris enlarges after menopause.

What men and women have in common during this critical midlife challenge is, first, the similarity in age at which it occurs (women may start a few years earlier, but in most couples the woman is a few years younger) and, second, the common suffering of serious emotional consequences. This commonality makes it even more important that the problem not be swept under the rug, as it so often has been in the past. I believe strongly that many a midlife divorce of an apparently otherwise happy couple can be avoided by dealing with this menopausal crisis honestly and directly.

4. Occasional Difficulties with Erections

In a study of over 1,500 men between the ages of 40 and 70, the Massachusetts Male Aging Study found that over half these individuals suffered from persistent problems with their erections. As these men aged from 40 to 70 years, there was a consistent increase in the number of men who had erectile difficulties at least half the time. How many of these men were additionally affected by the emotional consequences of male menopause is impossible to determine, but the number is probably larger rather than smaller. Clearly, sexual problems related to male menopause are not a rare occurrence.

5. Personality Changes

According to Dr. Karen Horney, there are three types of personalities: *towards* people, *against* people, and *away from* people. In other words, those who are people pleasers, those who are predominantly hostile, and those who seek refuge in withdrawal from others. According to the Massachusetts study, male menopause affects each of these types differently. The "people pleasers" ended up feeling intimidated and unable to make decisions; the hostile types ended up either bottling up their hostility or expressing it in full anger; the withdrawn types ended up depressed.

6. Denial

The saddest part of this whole phenomenon is the denial aspect. Since male menopause is not a socially accepted entity, and since most men and their mates are fairly ignorant of its manifestations, it turns out to cause so much more pain than is necessary. If this chapter does nothing more than educate you, your partner, and some close, supportive friends, then it's achieved its purpose in improving your life. By reducing the stress involved, your physical and emotional well-being are enhanced and a contribution is made to ten additional years of living longer and looking younger. In addition, if an understanding of male menopause can prevent any divorce action, then all the stress related to divorce is thus avoided, again adding to longer life and love.

7. Occurs only Once

Some people think that there may not be much difference between male menopause and a man's midlife crisis. Indeed, what is the difference?

For one thing, a man can have more than one midlife crisis. He may have one every 5 or 10 years or so, precipitated by some isolated challenge in his life. Male menopause, however, is much more likely to occur only once and it interconnects with a number of issues in his life, with such concerns as declining sexuality or the aging process in general as the main theme. It's also connected to the definite awareness of passing from a youth-oriented self-concept to one of accepting maturity and the inevitable lifestyle changes that are now imminent. Whereas midlife crisis can be a passing phase based on a single-issue challenge, male menopause is a psychological/ medical syndrome which is experienced as a passage of the spirit from one way of being to an entirely different, more thoughtful way of living life.

CONQUERING THE CHALLENGES OF THE MIDDLE YEARS

The emotional challenge of these middle years has to do primarily with a fearful anxiety combined with diminished self-esteem. As I mentioned earlier, there are three possible responses to this: repressed or fully-expressed hostility, depression, or a sense of being so overwhelmed that there is a loss of any decision-making ability.

Feelings of sexual inadequacy come into play precisely because of this dysfunction of emotions. Since it's normal to experience some decrease in sex drive somewhere between the ages of 40 and 60, this normal decrease can easily be interpreted by the menopausal male as an exaggerated sense of loss of virility. The consequent anxiety due to this apparent loss of virility can then cause a real loss of erectile potential, which causes more anxiety in this vicious cycle of downward-spiraling self-esteem. Anxiety diminishes sex drive, which in turn leads to greater fear of impotence, and so on. Herein is planted the seed of many a male menopause situation. What was a normal decrease in sex drive, very slight over a twenty-year period, has turned into a real case of male menopause-related impotence.

As if to reassure himself that he still appears youthful to the world despite his impotence, the menopausal male rushes to the mirror to appraise what remains of his youthful countenance, and what does he see? A more pronounced set of crow's feet, a few more gray hairs at his temples, a new discolored spot on the side of his face. To make sure, he reaches for a magnifying glass, hoping these signs of age will disappear under closer scrutiny. Instead, these dastardly signs of aging multiply in size and clarity, adding the insult of aging to the injury of impotence. As he looks out through the window beside the mirror into the blue sky above, he sees a plane skywriting in large, white letters, his full name. Underneath his name, two words: OLD FART.

Elizabeth Kubler-Ross described the stages one goes through in accepting loss: rejection, anger, acceptance, adjustment. And so it is with the loss of a youthful self-concept. The male menopause begins to be healed when rejection and anger no longer work. Then the task becomes acceptance and adjustment.

The mate of the menopausal male needs to be particularly sensitive at this stage. If ever the man needed to be taken care of, this is it. This is the time for a man's mate to prove her mettle as trustworthy and dependable. Male menopause results in the kind of stress that avoids resolution without outside help. A caring partner and, when feasible, an understanding psychotherapist are essential to coming to grips with male menopause.

Without such assistance, the menopausal male may continue to distort reality, exaggerating his loss of vigor as an unyielding obstacle. He may fall into deeper depression resulting in increasing irritability and withdrawal.

Who's to Blame?

When a successful man is his 50s discovers his own impotence with his wife after years of sexual fulfillment taken for granted, who is to blame? How does he account for it? Not understanding the basics of male menopause, his first reaction might be to focus on the lack of passion in his marriage and hope to achieve peace of mind only by focusing on an erotic younger partner. Divorce may be the only solution that he allows himself in order to maintain his male pride. But a more realistic, longer-lasting solution is to be found elsewhere—in a deeper understanding of the challenge of the male menopause.

The Grieving Process

Acceptance leads to a subsequent period of grieving, as I've mentioned, and that's a normal process. Loss requires grieving and grieve he must if the menopausal male is to move on to a healthy acceptance of his new role, with sufficient support from spouse and/or close friends and receptivity to professional counseling when necessary.

Acknowledgment and Support

Another important step in overcoming the crisis of male menopause is the public acknowledgement that such a phenomenon occurs. As I've mentioned earlier, Americans are more resistant than Europeans in accepting this as a common malady. If we could accept it as a common experience among middle-aged men, there would be less loneliness and pain among such men and their partners. A support group of men with or without their partners could be a very constructive means of overcoming the loneliness of male menopause.

Treating the Body with Respect

First of all, the midlife transformation from youth to maturity can be accepted for what it is—not a failure of the body, but rather a settling into a new physical lifestyle. Activities that involve quick jumps and starts along with expecting the muscles to respond with full capacity at a second's notice are no longer as appropriate. Instead men can look forward to a new respect for the body, accepting gradual challenges with more routine built into them. A greater awareness of his history of successes and failures in the gym and on the playing field can help determine future goals to build a stronger body with increasing stamina. What men took for granted till now must be treated with thoughtful consideration of how to make the best of what they have left. Yes, life is a limited commodity. As they come to appreciate its decreasing supply—as they must come to accept their own mortality—they learn to appreciate what they have left and treat it with the respect it deserves.

Becoming a Greater Lover

Second, and at least equally important, is the opportunity—at last!—to become a greater lover, particularly because such men no longer take the mechanics of sex for granted. They now have the opportunity to allow a greater appreciation of the more romantic and emotional nuances of sex to come into play.

Third, but not least, they can now attend to the greater complexity of the female sexual response more easily. Women have always wanted their men to pay attention to that, but many might have chosen to ignore it until now. Here's your chance to create a more satisfying experience for the both of you.

PLANNING AHEAD: OVERCOMING THE PROBLEMS OF MALE MENOPAUSE

1. Facing Reality

Regaining an accurate sense of perspective is the first step in overcoming the ravages of male menopause. Taking stock of your life, including your marital relationship, career, and financial security, with a healthy perspective, can be attained with the support of an understanding mate, intimate friends, or a professional counselor. Lifelong goals may need reshaping. The relative importance of financial vs. emotional priorities may need to be rearranged. It's likely that financial and career goals may need to be lowered to allow for the priority of family closeness and personal health. Whatever the shift, allow yourself a new openness to the fluidity of shifting priorities, so that your deeper needs are not pushed aside for more externally-reinforced values such as career success and accumulation of wealth.

There's nothing wrong with career success and wealth, except when they're attained at the sacrifice of physical and emotional health.

2. Becoming More Honest with Yourself

Facing the reality of aging and the inevitable decline in physical and sexual prowess may be painful at first, especially if denial has been going on for a while, but, once done, it allows for a refreshing acceptance of the inevitabilities of life. Focus on self can then gradually be replaced by an emotionally enriching process of supporting others, particularly those who can benefit—children, co-workers, proteges, younger friends. Personal goals can now be broadened to include the successes of other individuals. These relationships grow in depth so that others' successes can become as enriching as selfish success once was.

Instead of seeing a decline in your powers to influence others, you can come through this menopausal crisis now beginning to feel an undreamed-of sense of benevolent power. You can tap the vast storehouse of your knowledge and skills to enrich the lives of those who love and respect you.

3. Taking a Break

In order to shift priorities and make intelligent decisions that really work well and last over the years, a break in life's routine is essential. This is the time to take that relaxing and well-deserved vacation that's been postponed continually. If that's not possible, a relaxed, day-long drive in the countryside alone or with a loved one or understanding, intimate friend, may do the trick. Get away from the routine and give yourself an opportunity to reflect on your shift in priorities. If you've chosen to do that alone, then make sure to discuss your thoughts and resolutions with that special individual when you return.

4. Becoming an Expert in Sexual Foreplay

Although your mate is becoming more sexual, she may share with you the need for more foreplay. For some, female lubrication occurs more slowly after menopause, just as you might require more tactile stimulation to get aroused as the years go by. Talk, experiment, and explore till you find what works best for your mate. Communicate with one another using both words and hand guidance so that each of you becomes the world expert on turning the other on. This way, your sexual life becomes richer and more fulfilling even though your hormones are not raging as they were in your 20s. The hormones are still there; you just have to call them up.

5. Becoming an Expert in Afterplay

How would you feel about the opportunity to become a greater lover? Part of being a wonderful lover, beyond foreplay and sexual skills, is a component hardly ever mentioned: *afterplay.*

Afterplay is what happens after orgasm, lying together enjoying the enveloping experience of intimacy through loving words or undisturbed quiet, while romantic music continues in the background. Afterplay is cuddling and kissing, caressing and gentle massage, sometimes with your penis still inside her vagina. Afterplay is enjoying the setting together, be it starry sky and moonlight, or the city horizon through the window, or the fireplace.

Afterplay can also take place once you get out of bed (or off the kitchen table or wherever). It can involve sharing a nude jump in your private pool or a gentle foot massage. Afterplay can be sharing some special foods such as strawberries in champagne, wine from the same glass or an opulent feast, prepared beforehand, which you feed to one another in silence.

It really doesn't matter what form afterplay takes as long as it's done with warm, loving feelings. Generally, afterplay can involve holding, cuddling and love talk immediately afterwards, then bathing or gentle massage, and naturally enjoying the romantic aspects of the setting while favorite food or drink follow in soft candlelight.

Wham-bam-thank-you-Ma'am sex may work for 20-year-olds, but truly romantic loving is available throughout the rest of your lifespan. All it takes is the choice to become a greater lover. Coming out of male menopause is an excellent time to make that choice.

6. Exploring Spiritual Values

Whatever your spiritual or religious inclinations are, take stock of your spiritual side. We often become too preoccupied with the routine demands of daily life to reflect sufficiently on our spiritual needs.

Those individuals who live through their 80s and 90s typically reveal a strong spiritual component in their lives, which they've nurtured throughout their lives, not just in the senior years. As you accept your transformation from youth to maturity, spiritual awareness becomes more significant. During your 20s, you may have felt all-knowing and all-powerful. As you mature, life becomes more of a mystery and you may feel a more humble part of the complexity of life around you. As if to compensate as this shift occurs, there's also a growing respect for the unknown forces that seem to have a guiding force in making things work out in the end.

Those of you who have maintained a relationship with a church or temple are fortunate in having that community of friends and the rituals that are part of your religious experience. For those who have lost touch with such institutions, a spiritual awakening to your deeper feelings and lofty aspirations can enrich your understanding of the complexities of life. Freedom of thought and religious expression are too often taken for granted in Western democracies. If we only knew the pain and suffering (often torture and death) of those who express their thoughts and beliefs in some nondemocratic countries, we wouldn't take such freedoms for granted. Coming out of male menopause, you have the total freedom to explore and experiment with your spiritual values to find what holds the most meaning for you as you embark on the more deeply fulfilling half of your life.

7. Taking Control of Health Through Smart Eating and Fitness

Many men going through male menopause are close to their prime of life in terms of strength, vigor, and appearance. This is an excellent time to take control of eating habits to maintain a healthy weight. By gradually taking on an enjoyable set of physical fitness activities, whatever strength exists can be maintained and even increased over the coming years and decades. By taking control of your lifestyle with regard to eating and fitness, you can become more vital, healthier, and even more attractive. In the chapters to follow, many suggestions are offered to make all this possible. It's simply a matter of taking control.

8. An Understanding of Female Menopause

What better companion to weather this crisis than your own partner in life who is probably going through a similar crisis at somewhat the same time (give or take a few years)! If you'd like her to understand your crisis, then you surely need to understand hers.

Although your mate may be becoming more sexual throughout menopause just as you're becoming more concerned about your own sexuality, the previous chapter has explained how to catch up with her so that you're both "floating down the river of life in the same boat," sexually speaking.

As you begin to take charge of your life in terms of better health and lifestyle, why not become partners in this venture? Subsequent chapters will outline how to modify your eating habits, and explained why fitness will help you live longer and stay sexier for that longer lifespan. These suggestions work just as well for women as they do for men, so you can do much of it together.

Both of you might need more support as you make this difficult transition in self-concept. Your relationship can be enhanced greatly if you understand some of the common psychological challenges of male and female menopause. Each of you can indulge the other more as you now take into consideration that you're in this together.

ENTERING YOUR SECOND PRIME

By age 60 a number of men are taking medications for high blood pressure, which often becomes problematic by that age. Those or other medications, such as certain tranquilizers, may have an adverse effect on sexuality.

By the time men reach what I call *Age-60-Settling*, sex begins to take on an entirely new meaning. Sex for the sake of conquest has long become a thing of the past. Sex has become more of a sensual, intimate experience that brings back the romantic possibilities their female partners have longed for. Some become highly altruistic in the sense that they "get off" through their partner's orgasms. The sexual arousal may be somewhat slower and less intense, but the mind and body are strong enough to compensate by making great love instead of just having sex. And, occasionally, when things go just right, intensity of arousal for the male may be ecstatic and sublime, superior to anything he's had in his youth, as he brings all his senses and capacities to bear on the intimacy between himself and his partner.

Somewhere in the 50s, the male menopause brings one of life's greatest challenges to the fore. But a successful passage through that crisis can foster a wealth of riches in personal growth, including ways of combining sex with emotional intimacy. Only then can men reach for the highest levels of truly intimate sex, through their 60s, 70s, and even beyond.

Coming Through It with a Healthier Lifestyle

This second half of life has all the potential to be a fuller, more enjoyable one in every respect. As described elsewhere in this book, sex can be so much more satisfying to both partners. Eating can be healthier, and one can learn to become a gourmet (one who has finesse and panache) rather than a gourmand (one who is concerned with mere quantity). With more thoughtfulness, other aspects of lifestyle such as healthier sleeping and eating patterns, sensible exercise schedules, and sufficient time set aside for relaxation and family time can not only add a sense of control over and enjoyment of, life but also contribute to ten more years of living and loving younger.

The aging process, in a physical, sometimes sexual sense, is the key issue in male menopause. Therefore, physical exercise is one of the primary responses as a solution. The cardiovascular system is the most sensitive in terms of its effect on the aging process. When the blood stops flowing to any part of the body, that part dies, whether it's a section of the heart as in heart attack, a part of the brain as in stroke, a limb as in diabetes, or the penis as in impotence. Yes, the primary cause of impotence is insufficient flow of blood to the penis. So if you need any more encouragement to get up and exercise, to keep your circulatory system young and fit, to keep your body mean and lean, then read the following chapters of the book with special attention.

The next chapter, for a change of pace, will get you prepared to take the best advantage of useful nutritional information and offers suggestions on how to keep yourself healthy through use of adequate vitamin and mineral supplements to enhance your chances of living ten years longer. You'll learn how to assume a confident attitude by taking charge of your eating habits, learn how to master the skills of dining out in healthy fashion, so that you may maintain a healthy lifestyle that enables you to love ten years "younger" and live ten years longer.

You've already learned how to think young, how to keep young sexually, and how to motivate yourself to stay young through the middle years. In the remainder of this book, you'll learn how to keep your heart young and healthy, how to give up smoking if you haven't yet done so, and how to fine-tune your appearance. Looking ten years younger has two components: The first is made up of a combination of wise choices and health habits. That will be dealt with in chapter nine of this book. The second involves a strong, healthy attitude maintained by self-mastery. That's what we'll discuss in chapter eleven of this book.

This body of knowledge will not only give you ten more years of youthful appearance; it will give you ten more years of happier and more successful living as well.

DR. RYBACK'S
ANTIAGING FOOD PLAN

Eating is something most of us do at least three times a day. If we are in control of this ongoing activity, we can do more to look younger and live longer than any other single activity in our lives. Almost on a daily basis, we read about more and more research findings that inform us of the importance of choosing the right foods.

THE NATURAL HEALING POWER IN FRUITS AND VEGETABLES

Recent reports indicate that just by eating a couple of generous servings of such vegetables as carrots and broccoli and such fruits as apricots and cantaloupe, we can:

1. help avoid cancer;
2. decrease the risk of developing angina; and
3. prevent coronary heart disease in general.

Not bad, just for eating our fruits and veggies. And best of all, no side effects.

So, you see, it doesn't take all that much effort. It's just a matter of educating yourself and making some wise choices. In this chapter, we'll explore the basics of intelligent nutrition along with vitamin and mineral supplements and back this up with sound research. The basics are very simple. And in all likelihood, you've heard some of it before. But here we bring it all together so that we can minimize the confusion and gain control over what we put in our mouths.

How Each Diet Makes You Fatter

As we lose weight through dieting, fat cells do not shrink in number but merely in size. Once we give up on our diet, those little fat cells soak up all the fat they can to regain their normal size and if we continue our fat intake beyond that, then additional fat cells will add to our bulk. It appears that we can *increase* the number of fat cells *easily* but we cannot *decrease* their number. This helps us understand how we get fatter and fatter with each successive diet.

So, even though diets promise—and can deliver—weight losses of four or more pounds per week, such diets are effective only for a week or so, and then cause either a very frustrating plateau or a rebound effect to sabotage any remaining ounces of motivation.

Take Bill for example. Bill was 200 pounds overweight, what some people would call "fat." A brilliant man, he was on a path to self-destruction. Unless he could lose a good deal of this weight, Bill would soon die. He had little time to lose.

Slowly, after beginning his consultation with me, he began to reduce his caloric intake and to take up exercise, first walking with increasing distance and then working out a bit at the local "Y." To reinforce his decision to become a thinner, healthier man, and his commitment to look ten years younger and live ten years longer, I shared the following guidelines with him.

10 ANTIAGING NUTRITION BASICS

My antiaging food plan demands complete commitment and a full realization and acceptance of the fact that, inevitably, there will be setbacks. To do it right, be absolutely sure you don't overlook the following ten basic rules:

1. Set Reasonable Goals

Be wary of standard height/ weight tables. What is really important is the ratio of muscle to fat. For instance, a very muscular individual may appear too fat according to some standard tables. And a man who is out of shape may appear to be the right weight, though he has the wrong muscle-to-fat ratio.

A more efficient standard for men would be for body fat to be 15 to 22 percent of total body weight. To best determine your body fat (other than with hydrodensitometry or underwater weighing), have someone with experience measure you with skin calipers. Try a good health club or your local university's department of physical education, exercise physiology, or nutrition.

2. Don't Lose Sight of Reality

Important: Slow and gradual weight loss works. Sudden and dramatic losses in weight don't work. The body needs to adjust to weight loss if the loss is to be even somewhat permanent. Ideally, you should plan to lose about one or two pounds per week. It's much better to take a year to lose 50 pounds and keep it off in a healthy manner than to impress yourself and others with a dramatic loss that just comes back to haunt you and shame you to your friends. Best of all, it's much easier to do it the healthier way.

The dramatic ads you see in the magazines and on TV to shed pounds quickly and effortlessly in weeks (or even days) are false and pernicious. The only part of your being that will end up permanently lighter will be your wallet. These ads take advantage of the fact that it is easy to lose weight in the beginning of any diet, but this is mainly due to water loss.

3. Convert Poor Nutritional Habits to Good Ones

Discover your patterns of eating by keeping an eating journal. For a couple of weeks, keep note of (1) what you eat, (2) how much, (3) when, (4) where, (5) what you're doing at the time, and (6) how you're feeling at the time.

The answers to these questions will help you discover the pattern of your eating habits. Only then will you learn how to change these patterns so that you can gain control over the details of your life that determine your particular eating habits.

You may be surprised how much certain places (restaurant, lounge), times (noon, dinner time), activities (watching sports on TV or movies), or feelings (frustration, anger) determine your eating habits. Instead of letting these circumstances decide, you can now master your eating habits by controlling some of these circumstances, at least some of the time. You can gain more control over these circumstances over time just as you can learn any other skill—with *attention* and *intention*.

4. Follow a Balanced, Low-Fat Food Plan

Make sure to eat a variety of foods from the basic food groups. Whenever possible, choose carbohydrates over fats. Eat lots of fruits, vegetables, and grains. This makes you feel full and provides good nutrition at a most reasonable cost.

5. Avoid High-Fat Foods

Do your best to avoid high-fat foods such as red meat and its by-products:

- ❐ hamburger, meat loaf
- ❐ hot dogs, luncheon meats

as well as:

- ❐ whole milk and cheese
- ❐ baked goods such as cookies, cakes, doughnuts
- ❐ fried foods
- ❐ gravy and cream sauce
- ❐ most crackers and chips
- ❐ ice cream
- ❐ most nuts, especially almond, macadamia, and coconut

6. Find the Eating Pattern That's Comfortable for You

The important thing here is to explore patterns of eating until you find one that feels comfortable for you and, more than that, gives you a sense of mastery over your eating habits and, consequently, your body weight. Otherwise, the changes you worked so hard to achieve will be short-lived.

7. Drink Water with a Squeeze of Lemon

Whatever option you choose, it is essential that you drink sufficient fluids throughout the day. It's a good idea to drink about eight cups of water throughout the day, even if you drink it in the form of your favorite beverages. Keep in mind, too, though, that many soft drinks contain hefty measures of sugar unless they are diet drinks. A squeeze of lemon in cool water is an excellent option.

8. Learn to Limit Libations

Limit your alcohol to no more than two drinks a day.

9. Exercise

The best insurance against regaining the weight you've lost is to incorporate exercise into your everyday routine.

Find an activity that you can (1) enjoy, (2) fit into your life so that you can continue it without too much difficulty, and (3) make sure that it's an ongoing part of your life by arranging the rest of your life around it.

Here are some helpful hints:

❏ Make a routine of your exercise activity but allow for interesting changes within that routine. For example, if swimming is your activity, you might vary the strokes. If jogging, you might vary the route or the type of music you enjoy on your Walkman. Or alternate your activities between swimming and jogging, if those are your activities of choice.

❏ Arrange your schedule so that you exercise the same time each day. That will help make it a permanent fixture in your life without your having to make a decision to exercise each time.

❏ If you enjoy exercising alone, you can choose from: walking, jogging, swimming, weight lifting, machine rowing, cycling, hitting a ball against a backboard, shooting baskets, and so on.

❐ If you prefer socializing, choose from any of the above with your favorite friends, or enjoy team sports such as tennis, basketball, soccer. Join the local Y and see what it has to offer. If you have a lot of social frustration in your life, you might consider judo or karate.

❐ If you drive to work, park a few blocks from work (which may save you parking fees). Walk the rest of the way to work and jog back to your car after work. Take the stairs instead of the elevator. Instead of having a three-course meal at the cafeteria, take a noontime stroll and finish it off with low-fat yogurt and fresh fruit. Then spend the rest of the afternoon enjoying how much better you feel than your associates.

10. Create Meaningful Markers or Milestones to Celebrate Your Successes

For example, for each 5, 10, or 20 pounds you lose, reward yourself with something you enjoy but wouldn't ordinarily give yourself. A ticket for a playoff game, taking a close friend to one of your favorite restaurants to share a healthy meal, buying yourself an article of clothing you've wanted or a special watch—any of these can be an exciting reward to be anticipated to help motivate your thinner self.

POWER BREAKFAST FOR LASTING YOUTH

According to one study at The VA Medical Center in Minneapolis, when 14 volunteers were given free rein at a buffet of munchies and snack foods, those who had eaten the highest-fiber cereal for breakfast ate about 45 calories less at the buffet three and a half hours later.

A follow-up study divided volunteers into two groups. One had very high- and the other very low-fiber cereal for breakfast. At the buffet, later in the day, the high-fiber group chose to eat 90 calories less than the other group. Moral: Starting the day with high-fiber cereal (with skim milk, of course) gives you a great head start. This one small step in itself with no other changes, continued over the span of a year, could result in a 10-pound weight loss.

Lasting youth and health, according to the National Academy of Sciences, is helped by at least five daily servings of vegetables and fruits, especially green and yellow vegetables and citrus fruits. The Department of Health and Human Services recommends even more—as many as eight servings. So a good start at breakfast to get your share of power foods is most important.

In addition to high-fiber cereal with skim milk, consider fresh fruit juice, with a cup of cottage cheese or low-fat yogurt containing some fresh fruit such as banana or pineapple. If you enjoy waffles or pancakes, top them with sliced fruit instead of syrup.

If you have no time for a sit-down breakfast, at least start your day off with a blended fruit smoothie. Try banana along with one or two other fruits for the luxurious but low-fat creamy texture that the banana will give to it.

Another fast-breakfast idea comes all the way from China. The Chinese take rice left from the previous evening's meal and, using water, create a healthy, soup-like cereal. If you want to add more power to this exotic breakfast dish, add some sesame seeds and bits of cooked chicken or fish.

FOODS THAT MAKE YOU OLD

Moving beyond breakfast, and taking a general overview, the worst foods, those to avoid as much as possible, fall into four main categories:

1. Red meat and its by-products—hamburgers, cheeseburgers, meatloaf.
2. Processed meats such as hot dogs, ham, and lunch meats.
3. Whole milk and cheese (except for low-fat cheese and yogurts).
4. Baked goods such as cookies, cakes, and doughnuts.

These foods are major sources of total fat, generally included in the American diet. Remember, too much fat in your body is implicated in certain cancers, diabetes, hypertension, digestive problems, and complications in arthritis, not to mention heart disease and high serum cholesterol.

One of the factors responsible for meat making you old is the manner in which it is cooked or preserved. The way that hot dogs are cured, for example, contributes to cancer. Browned—or worse, charred—meats are known to contribute to cancer as well.

The frying or broiling of meats creates carcinogens both within the meat, and on the more apparent surface. Such carcinogens tend to form throughout the meat's outer third.

Another category of food that makes you old is that of processed, prepackaged microwave-ready meals. They are usually high in calories with little fiber content. They typically (but not always) provide 30 percent or more calories from fat. They are almost always high in sodium content, as well.

Finally, a tricky category of food that makes you old: any packaged food that is labeled in some healthy fashion, yet makes you old in some hidden way. Sound confusing? That's the advertisers' intent.

Some examples: 2 percent milk can be advertised as "low-fat milk," yet it may keep us from choosing skim milk, which *does* have the power to keep us younger and healthier. Prepackaged luncheon meals may boast "lean chicken" and "lean turkey," but the whole combination with cheese included comes to a very high fat level. So take those "healthy" come-ons with a grain of suspicion.

HOW FRESH FRUITS AND VEGETABLES ADD YEARS TO YOUR LIFE

According to the ongoing Framingham Heart Study, those who eat little fat will live almost two years longer than those who eat fatty foods. Clearly, eating healthy contributes to living longer.

Beyond vitamins and minerals, fiber and carbohydrates, there's a newly recognized substance that can add years to your life: *phyto-*

chemicals. These are instrumental in helping to prevent the onset of cancer, and are stored by the hundreds in most plant foods. As a result of this discovery, the medical community is becoming more appreciative of the healthy nature of a vegetarian style of eating. More and more doctors are understanding the capacity of fruits and vegetables to add healthy years to your life.

Over 12 million Americans now consider themselves vegetarians, but within this large group are smaller groupings, based on the degree of dedication to this style of nutrition. Here's how they break down.

Most of these 12 million fall into the category known as *semivegetarians*. They eat no red meat for the most part, but occasionally eat chicken and other fowl, or fish.

Lacto-ovo-vegetarians eat no meat at all, not even fowl, but will eat animal products, such as milk and eggs, unlike the *lacto-vegetarians* who eat no eggs, or the *vegans* who eat no eggs and no milk products.

Many in the larger group who consider themselves vegetarians will nonetheless eat red meat, but very occasionally, and work toward minimizing their consumption of any kind of meat or fish. This seems to be the trend in society at large—toward less meat and more fruit and vegetables, at least among those who are mindful of adding years to their lives.

How to Fill Yourself Up and Still Stay Thin

You could probably eat much more than you do now without gaining weight if there were no fat or sugar in the foods you did eat. Such foods as fruits and vegetables and whole wheat foods free of fat would likely fill you up before they'd make you fat. The Food Guide Pyramid recommends a daily intake of 6 to 11 servings of some combination of bread, cereal, rice, or pasta; 2 to 4 servings of fruit; 3 to 5 servings of vegetables; and lesser servings of the other food groupings, with a sparing use of fats, oils, and sweets. This guide, released by the U.S. Dept. of Agriculture, is a marked reduction from the previous years' recommendations for meat and dairy product amounts.

The "Protein Myth"

The problem with animal protein is that it is high in artery-clogging saturated fat and cholesterol. Besides that, most men eat more protein than they need anyway. Adult American men eat about 30 percent more, in fact.

Furthermore, it may come as a surprise to most of you that you don't need *any* animal protein to be healthy. You can get all the protein you need from nonmeat sources. Yet many "red-blooded" Americans (whatever that means) think they need to have a steak a day to eat properly. Americans eat an average of 10.6 ounces of red meat a day compared to the 2.24 ounces eaten daily by the Japanese, to use one comparison.

Finding Low-Fat Meats

For those men who have to have their dole of red meat, there are some interesting options coming up. Buffalo meat gets only 15 percent of its calories from fat. If Ted Turner and Jane Fonda are successful in making buffalo meat more popular, we may be seeing more of it. Further down the line is the possibility of ostrich meat, another relatively low-fat "red" meat. In the meantime, keep in mind that it has been shown in scientific studies that mice fed 40 percent less red meat than their counterparts have lived twice as long.

The Magic of Drinking Water

This might be a good point to remind you of the benefits of drinking six to eight glasses of water each day. The older we get, the more important this becomes. As we mature, we hold less cellular water, 10 to 15 percent less by age 65. More water will certainly help us look younger as our skin cells enjoy the liquid refreshment along with all other cells.

STAY YOUNG WITH A HIGH-FIBER, LOW-FAT DIET

Losing weight with minimal deprivation can be best accomplished not by counting calories, or by measuring out small food portions but rather by committing yourself to a high-fiber, low-fat style of eating.

Earlier, you read about the trend toward vegetarian-style eating. Medical research is proving this to be the most effective, longest-lasting approach to weight loss and staying younger.

It's not how much you eat that matters. Different men need differing amounts of food. What does matter is the *quality* of the food you eat, in terms of fat and fiber. By following the suggestions you've read so far in this chapter, you're on your way to staying younger. By avoiding high-fat meats (especially fried) and milk products (especially cheese on pizza, and cheesecake and ice cream), you're more likely to choose healthier vegetables, fruits, and grains. Not only will you look younger and live longer; you'll feel better, too, with more energy and greater alertness.

Furthermore, it's much easier. Rather than having to make many small decisions about how much to deprive yourself of rich foods, you make a big decision only once: a decision to eat healthy foods. Instead of constantly being reminded of what you're missing, you learn to enjoy the healthy foods you're choosing.

A choice to eat this way automatically provides more fiber in your diet without your having to think about it. A breakfast of high-fiber cereal with skim milk topped with half a banana along with some orange juice will keep you satisfied until you can enjoy a mid-morning snack a couple of hours later. At this time you can treat yourself to whole-wheat toast or bagel with a bit of jam or jelly or, if you're at work, a piece of your favorite fruit. For lunch, you can enjoy some pasta with vegetables and salad, making sure that any sauces or dressings are of the very low-fat variety.

The simple thing to remember: the less processed, the better! Raw vegetables and fruits are best. Next in order: brown rice, high-fiber bread and cereal, potatoes (unhampered by butter, of course), and pasta. Fish is better than fowl, and fowl is better than red meat, which should not be marbled with fat. Skin on fowl should be avoided. (Choose white meat over dark meat, since the dark has twice as much fat as the white.)

What to Substitute

Instead of mayonnaise, try lettuce, tomato, or cucumber for moisture. Instead of potato chips, try unsalted pretzels or plain popcorn. Instead of ice cream, try ice milk or sorbet. And be careful of that innocent looking peanut butter—two tablespoons contain 16.2 grams of fat.

Right and Wrong Breads

Breads can be very healthy and enjoyable, especially "designer" breads flavored with lusty garlic and dill or onions and rosemary. Look for breads that are chewier and have big bubbles inside. They're the ones that tend to be fat-free. Avoid the ones that have a tender, cakey texture with tiny bubbles—they're full of fat. And if the bread itself is tasty, you don't need to add fatty condiments like butter or peanut butter. Ask for fat-free, whole wheat bread and you're more likely to get a healthy dose of fiber as well. If you don't go in for "designer" breads, then your best supermarket breads are Wonder High Fiber Wheat, Roman Meal Light Oat Bran 'N Honey or Roman Meal Light Seven Grain, each of which has no more than 1 gram of fat and about 6 grams of fiber per serving. Your worst choice, by far, would be Sara Lee Croissant, weighing in at 6 grams of fat and merely 0.1 grams of fiber per serving. So choose your bread carefully.

MORE CARBOS MEAN MORE ENERGY

Carl, a 51-year-old college professor of political science at a nearby university, had just gone through a midlife crisis and was determined to shed the extra pounds around his waist. He had just gone through an ugly divorce and because of his readings on environmental issues, he decided to give up meat.

"How," asked Carl, "can I continue to eat a well-balanced diet without meat? Do I need to take protein pills?"

"Of course not!" I reassured him, "You can get all the protein you need by combining beans, grains, and low-fat dairy products."

By now you can see the direction in which I'm pointing you. Animal foods such as meat and eggs and whole-milk products have no place in your diet once you make a choice to live ten years longer. Only modest portions of low-fat animal foods are to be included in your new eating habits: skinless chicken or turkey breast, fish, nonfat yogurt or cottage cheese, and skim milk. If you choose to avoid meat and fish altogether, then you can replace those with more complex carbohydrates, such as beans, peas, and lentils.

If you must eat meat, then your best choice of red meat is select beef tip or eye of round. Your best choice of seafood is baked or broiled flounder or sole. If you choose to eat pork, select tenderloin. If you must eat eggs, stick to egg whites or find an egg substitute to your liking.

For those who choose to give up meat, the choice of beans and grain becomes more important. Complex carbohydrates are close to being the perfect food for living ten years longer. They are the lowest fat-to-fiber-ratio foods around, giving you the most nutrition per calorie. Fresh fruits, vegetables, beans, and whole grains all are complex carbohydrates. We've already discussed fruits and vegetables. Now we'll focus on beans and grains.

Aside from being almost fat-free and full of fiber, beans and grains contain amino acids which combine to provide your body with protein. They also contain a number of vitamins and minerals. Here is an overview of what some common beans offer:

	Black Beans	Great Northern Beans	Kidney Beans	Navy Beans
B_6	0.1mg.	1mg.	0.2mg.	1mg.
Calcium	47mg.	90mg.	50mg.	95mg.
Fiber	7g.	9g.	6g.	9g.
Iron	4mg.	5mg.	5mg.	5mg.
Potassium	611mg.	750mg.	713mg.	790mg.

These also contain folic acid, magnesium, copper, zinc, manganese, and phosphorus.

For those who are concerned about intestinal gas which some experience from eating beans, there is a solution. Boiling the beans in a large saucepan with $1/8$ teaspoon of baking soda for 10 minutes prior to cooking will solve most of the problem. Allow the beans to cool and allow to soak at room temperature in the same water for 8 to 10 hours. Then discard the water and rinse before cooking as usual.

Another method is the simple use of the commercial product known as Beano, which, when added to bean dishes, converts the indigestible sugars into readily absorbed sugars. A free sample can be obtained by calling (800) 257–8650.

If you're not used to eating beans, start slowly, until your system adapts to them.

Just like beans, grains are also low in fat and high in fiber, at least before commercial refining. They can provide the source of ongoing, constant energy, since they are stored as glycogen in the muscles. They are eaten mostly in the form of bread, pasta, cereal, and rice dishes. Since they're low fat and filling, they do much to help you keep your weight down by providing an alternative to higher-fat foods.

Simply choose foods made up of whole grains rather than refined forms, and you're on your way. Whole-grain products provide insoluble fiber, which helps reduce the risk of colon cancer; and soluble fiber, which lowers blood cholesterol. Unfortunately, most of the grains available to Americans are the refined type. So it's important to learn more about whole grains (including their nutritious hulls and germs).

Among the most common and most nutritious in the U.S. is *whole-wheat flour* (as opposed to refined white flour). This grain can be found in whole-wheat bagels, breads, English muffins, pasta, waffles, and wheat-bran. *Bulgur,* wheat that has been dried and cracked, can be eaten as a cereal or side dish. Cracked-wheat salad, known as *tabbouleh,* can be a nutritious alternative to white rice.

Rice, the most common grain in the world, is most commonly consumed in the U.S. in its refined, white, polished form, deprived of its protein, minerals, and B vitamins. *Whole-grain* or *brown rice* are clearly the more nutritious alternatives.

Rye, oats, and *buckwheat* can be consumed in their whole-grain form in breads. Pumpernickel bread is made with dark, coarse rye ground entirely from the kernel. Oats, barley, buckwheat, and rye can be consumed in the form of cooked cereal, as in *oatmeal, barley soup, kasha*, and *porridge*, respectively.

A relatively unknown but rising star among healthy grains is *quinoa* (pronounced keen-wah). The most nutritious of all grains, quinoa contains all eight amino acids, is high in vitamin A and is one of the most protein-packed grains on the planet. It can be eaten in soups, stews, pilafs and bread to which it has been added.

If you're truly committed to living ten years longer, then you can't ignore grains as a principal nutrient in your dietary lifestyle. In addition to eating them as ingredients in other dishes, you can also learn to cook them and then just mix with a favorite flavor or topping. Generally, 1 cup of grain simmered in liquid will yield 2 to $3^1/_2$ cups cooked.

Other ways of eating grains consist of sprinkling cooked grains onto salads, or into stews or soups. Whole wheat, brown rice, or quinoa can be substituted for pasta dishes for a change of pace.

The new Food Guide Pyramid recommends six servings if you don't exercise and nine to eleven servings if you do exercise. So most of us need at least twice as much as was previously recommended by nutritionists. Here are some simple ways of increasing your intake of grains:

1. Instead of high-fat snacks such as cookies or candy bars, try air-popped popcorn or rice cakes.

2. Instead of a little pasta with lots of high-fat Alfredo sauce, try more pasta with low-fat marinara sauce.

3. Allow yourself thick slabs of whole-grain bread with low-fat topping instead of thin slices of bread covered with high-fat toppings.

4. Instead of one sandwich with high-fat meat or cheese, take the luxury of two or three sandwiches with whole-wheat bread stuffed with leafy greens, tomatoes, and cucumbers.

These complex-carbohydrate treats will fill you up with healthy nutrients without getting you fatted up. It's one of the secrets of getting thinner and healthier without depriving yourself. You get to enjoy your food, have more energy, and live longer in better health.

Eating Out and Staying Thin

Whenever I eat out, I'm overwhelmed by the choices of entrées with heavy and fattening creams, gravies, and sauces. As a single male I eat out quite often, and each time I'm confronted with the same dilemma: how to enjoy my meal without yielding to fat that might rob me of my ten extra years. Here are the results of years of personal experimentation and a reading of recent research in nutrition.

When you eat out, you can make certain choices that will minimize fats and increase the proportion of healthier foods. Here's what to do for various ethnic restaurants.

Chinese: Order steamed fish and rice or scallops sauteed with vegetables instead of with heavy sauces.

Mexican: Order steamed instead of fried tortillas. In your better restaurants, try red snapper Vera Cruz. Avoid dishes loaded with cheese or heavy sauces. Avoid fried rice.

French: Order grilled or poached fish or chicken breast with steamed vegetables, along with salade Nicoise with low-fat dressing on the side. Avoid heavy sauces, no matter how tempting. Instead of pastry for dessert, order fresh fruit.

Italian: Order pasta dishes with marinara (meatless) sauce rather than fat-laden Alfredo. Order baked chicken rather than high-fat cheese-laden pizza.

Men can have fun eating out and still stay healthy. It just involves making the right choices to stay thinner and live longer.

EATING FOR YOUTHFUL FLEXIBILITY

For healthy bones and flexibility, most men need about 25 percent more calcium than they typically get. Older men can be subject to the same problems of osteoporosis from which women are more commonly known to suffer. Men lose about one fifth of their bone mass over the course of a lifetime. Men who get more calcium in their diet suffer from fewer hip fractures.

Calcium for Healthy Bones and Blood Pressure

Calcium is found primarily in milk and dairy products. Since many men suffer from lactose intolerance and don't drink milk, it's important to get this vital mineral through supplementation. Calcium may also be useful in keeping our blood pressure normal.

Calcium, in the form of milk, has had a reputation for having mild "tranquilizing" effects for generations, though there are no scientific data to bear this out. A number of studies do, however, point to the importance of calcium for normalizing blood pressure.

Since I recommend a diet very high in fruits, vegetables, and carbohydrates (i.e., low-calorie, high-fiber), calcium is particularly important. Although I recommend a daily intake of 1 gram, a daily intake of up to 2 or 3 grams is quite safe. Incidentally, part of my calcium supplementation is in the form of Tums™ fruit-flavored antacid tablets, which have a very pleasant, candy-like taste and texture. I definitely don't have stomach problems—I just enjoy that safe, pleasant form of calcium carbonate.

Calcium strengthens bones more efficiently when accompanied by adequate amounts of vitamin D. Aside from exposure to sunlight, vitamin D can be obtained from fish and fortified milk. Those men who live high in the northern hemisphere where sunlight is relatively weak in the wintertime and who, at the same time, may not get sufficient amounts of fish and fortified milk, can benefit from a daily supplement of 400 International Units of vitamin D.

The U.S. Food and Drug Administration recommends a daily intake of 1000 mg. of calcium. The best source is food rather than supplements, and the foods that supply calcium are dairy products (skim milk, yogurt, fat-free mozzarella cheese), fish and shellfish, fruits, vegetables, grains, and beans.

Each of the following foods will supply about 300 mg. of calcium:

2 cups of cottage cheese

2 cups of ice milk

5 oz. of salmon

8 oz. of skim milk

1 cup of yogurt

In a typical day, you can easily ensure your youthful flexibility by treating yourself to a couple of glasses of skim milk, a cup of beans, some whole-wheat cereal, a cup of non-fat yogurt, and 3 oz. of fish (not necessarily in that order).

If, for whatever reason, you choose to take supplements instead, there are both chewable and nonchewable tablets available; there are many varieties as well. The least expensive chewables cost less than $2 per month. It's best to take calcium supplements with meals or at bedtime for best absorption. One thing to watch out for is taking calcium supplements with iron pills or multivitamins containing iron, since calcium interferes with iron absorption.

POWER FOODS FOR LASTING YOUTH

Any food that fortifies the immune system is one that I would consider to be a "power food." With a stronger immune system, your body can more easily defend itself against aging ravages of bacterial and viral infection as well as against dreaded cancer.

Your defense system is made up of certain "policing" cells—including B-cells, T-cells, and natural killer (NK) cells—that engulf and destroy cancer cells and infecting agents. When viruses, bacteria, or cancer cells start invading your body, it is the B-cells that produce the antibodies to fight against them. You may have heard of the natural substance called *interferon*, which helps fight against cancer. Well, this is produced by the T-cells. The NK cells help to fight against cancer and viral infections, too.

Power Food I: Delicious Yogurt

Yogurt has earned a fine reputation over the years as a "folk medicine" that keeps older people young. Now there's scientific evidence that it may do so by enhancing the immune function. Cultures existing in regular yogurt increase the amount of interferon in the immune system by a factor of five. Eating only two cups of yogurt daily for a period of four months will give you this added advantage.

Recent research has shown that yogurt enhances the power of NK cells to ward off cancer, particularly lung and colon cancer.

Power Food II: Tasty Garlic

Most of you have also heard of the supposed healing effects of garlic. It does enhance the functioning of the immune system, most specifically by stimulating the potency of T-cells.

If you don't like the effect of garlic on your social life, have no fear. You can get the same effect from odor-free garlic extract. This will make your NK cells at least twice as powerful as those who avoid garlic.

Power Food III: Asian Shiitake Mushrooms

You'll most often find these deliciously prepared delicacies at Chinese restaurants, nestling among other exotic vegetables. But whether you eat them there or prepare them at home yourself, these wonderful mushrooms, according to a series of research studies, contain a substance called *lentinal*, which significantly increases the number of T-cells as well as the production of other cancer-fighting substances.

Lentinal can also prevent the spreading of lung cancer cells. So this exotic mushroom not only helps reduce your risk of cancer; it helps stop it from spreading as well.

Power Food IV: Beta-carotene in Fruits and Vegetables

Although there may be some controversy about beta-carotene as a supplement, there is no disagreement about the powerful qualities of this substance found in natural foods and its ability to keep you younger. The controversy about the supplement form has to do with the difficulty in isolating the effective forms of the substance. However, when you get it by eating fruits and vegetables, you get all the forms of the substance that nature intends you to get so your body can enjoy its youth-enhancing properties.

Enjoy your share of such naturally sweet foods as sweet potatoes, carrots, pumpkin, as well as spinach, and you'll get enough beta-carotene to get more powerful NK cells and an immune system with twice the power.

The ability of this power food to keep you younger is even more important as you reach maturity, when the immune system starts to decline with the years. A mere 60 mg. of beta-carotene daily results in a significant increase in the percentage of NK cells and T-cells.

Power Food V: Foods Containing the Minerals Copper and Zinc

Both copper and zinc help keep the immune system operating at full efficiency, building strong defenses through T-cells and antibodies.

Once we reach middle age, the thymus gland begins to shrink and reduce its output of thymulin. This reduction becomes significantly marked after age 60. Daily low doses of zinc can result in as much as 80 percent regrowth of the thymus gland with significant increases in the number of T-cells. When 15 mg. of zinc per day were supplied to a group of individuals over the age of 65, their T-cell activity was as efficient as that of much younger people.

Power foods containing copper are dried peas and beans, fruits, and shellfish. Those containing zinc are cereals, beans, turkey, and oysters.

All these power foods contain building blocks that keep the immune system from aging, thereby helping to maintain a healthier, more attractive body ten more years.

YOUTH-BUILDING VITAMINS AND MINERALS

Vitamin and mineral supplements can help us live longer. We're better off getting these substances directly from the food sources, but most of us can't count on eating enough of the right amounts of such foods all the time. So supplements are for insurance so that, just in case we're not getting all our vitamins directly from the food sources, we're sure to get them in supplement form. As such they're relatively inexpensive, relatively safe from side effects and a form of health maintenance that we can control easily. Supplements are one of the tickets to ride to ten more years of healthy, attractive living.

Taking the regimen of vitamins and minerals recommended in this chapter will help you live ten years longer, live more comfortably, and look more attractive by helping to:

1. Avoid the onset of various types of cancers.

2. Decrease the risk of heart and circulatory diseases.

3. Lower cholesterol levels.

4. Improve circulation.

5. Slow down the aging process through antioxidants.

6. Promote the effective functioning of your immune system.

7. Protect against environmental pollution and food additives.

8. Fight viral infections.

9. Prevent anemia.

10. Detoxify harmful substances.

11. Rid the body of poisonous metals such as mercury and cadmium.

12. Alleviate symptoms and disabilities of rheumatoid arthritis.

13. Reduce your craving for sweets, thereby helping you to lose weight (see section on chromium picolinate).

14. Keep your skin healthy.

Vitamins Prolong Life

Naturally occurring substances in your diet can help prevent the "rusting" or aging process. The most common of these elements are the vitamins C, E, and beta-carotene, and minerals such as selenium and zinc. Although these substances do occur naturally in our diets, they may not be in sufficient quantity to prolong our lives as much as we'd like.

VITAMIN C: LINUS PAULING'S PROMISE OF (ALMOST) ETERNAL YOUTH

In his lifetime, Dr. Linus Pauling clearly spent more time researching the benefits of vitamin C than any other human being on this planet. He was unequivocally a strong advocate of its benefits and had written a good deal to substantiate his claims. Although the conventional regimen for vitamin C recommended by nutritionists is about 60 mg. per day, Pauling himself ingested 18 grams (18,000 mg.!) each and every day of his adult life. But Dr. Pauling didn't recommend that for everyone.

Pauling stressed very strongly that each individual has a unique biochemistry that calls for different amounts of vitamin C, ranging from as little as one quarter of a gram a day to 20 or more grams per day. So how do you discover your own optimal regimen?

First of all, you must begin by realizing that vitamin C is one of the very few substances that cannot seriously harm you if ingested in large quantities. Research has shown that even an equivalent of 350 grams (350,000 mg.) a day will not be very harmful. What does happen is that when you reach your optimal dosage, anything beyond that will cause diarrhea. That's nature's subtle way of telling you when you've reached your optimal dosage. When you reach that point, you merely scale back a bit until you regain normalcy once again. Vitamin C is virtually nontoxic. But, more specifically, what can vitamin C, at optimal dosage, do to extend your lifespan?

A Skeptical Doctor Is Converted

Vitamin C is best known as a cold fighter. One skeptic was Dr. Sherry Lewin, head of the Department of Molecular Biology at London Polytechnic. Experimenting on himself, Dr. Lewin tried taking 50 mg. of C per day. This didn't seem to do much. Dr. Lewin was on the verge of resuming his strong criticism of vitamin C. Then, one day, his wife came home with the only form of C she could find during her daily shopping—1 gram in an effervescent tablet. Not wanting to waste these tablets, Dr. Lewin took two or three of these each day and, to his surprise, found that the "incidence, severity, and duration" of his bad colds were greatly reduced. He then got the cooperation of 69 of his colleagues in testing the vitamin and the results indicated a better than 90 percent improvement rate.

Encouraged by this surprising finding, Lewin then went on to research the biological reasons for this and ended up writing and publishing a book. Dr. Lewin's primary finding was that there are different needs for C in different individuals. Robert Cathcart, an orthopedic surgeon, substantiated the diarrhea factor for discovering individual optimal dosages of C. As a matter of fact, Cathcart believes that unless C is taken at optimal dosage for a given individual, desirable effects should not be expected. If that's true, no wonder there's so much debate about the effectiveness of vitamin C.

How Vitamin C Adds Years to Life

Since colds rarely kill us, how can vitamin C extend our lifespan? The answer to that lies in the fact that vitamin C plays a much more major role in our bodies than in just helping us resist colds. Thousands and thousands of published scientific papers all point to the pervasive effect of vitamin C on all the physiological processes going on within our bodies. A brief summary for vitamin C—It:

1. plays a very important role in the health of our heart and its entire vascular system;

2. can play a very important role in the prevention and treatment of cancer;

3. promotes the healing of tissue wounds;

4. aids in the prevention of broken bones;

5. plays a very significant role in keeping our immune systems functioning in a healthy manner;

6. helps overcome male infertility;

7. counteracts the symptoms of asthma;

8. protects against smoking and various pollutants;

9. helps prevent diabetes, in terms of stabilizing sugar levels and energy metabolism.

Thirty-Five More Years?

This is not to say that vitamin C alone will extend your life span. Obviously, man does not live by C alone. Other vitamins and minerals as well as healthier lifestyle habits in general are necessary to live longer, more youthful lives. If we take charge of our diets and other habits, then we have a comprehensive grasp on controlling the length and quality of our lives. "My estimate, made on the basis of the results of epidemiological and other observations," said Dr. Pauling, "is that through the optimum use of vitamin supplements and other health measures, the length of the period of well-being and the length of life could be increased by twenty-five to thirty-five years."

At Least Ten More Years!

I'm a bit more modest. I'm just promising you ten more years of youthful, enjoyable life. I'd rather be conservative in what I hope for. But that's ten more years than you'd otherwise have.

What are the more important functions of the vitamins, in addition to what we've already discussed? Here are some answers, in alphabetical order.

Vitamin A Purifies the Blood

The chief function of *vitamin* A, stored in the liver, is the purification of the blood from such pollutants as pesticides, industrial poisons, and the toxic side effects of prescribed medications. It sometimes also retards the development of cancerous tumors. However, it is preferable to take beta-carotene, which is converted to vitamin A by the body as needed, and thereby avoids the possibility of overdosing on this fat-soluble vitamin.

Choose Niacin over Niacinamide

The reason I recommend the niacin form of B_3 (which causes flushing) over the niacinamide form (which doesn't) is because only niacin has been found to reduce cholesterol and triglyceride levels, perhaps even reversing atherosclerosis. Scientists researching this function of niacin claim that no other single agent has such potential for lowering both cholesterol and triglycerides. Take niacin after meals (as you should all vitamin pills) should reduce any flushing.

Other Essential Vitamins

Vitamin B_6 is one of the most important of the B vitamins. It:

1. protects against cancer,
2. helps keep the skin healthy, and
3. boosts the immune system.

Pantothenic acid is useful not only in alleviating the painful symptoms and disability of rheumatoid arthritis but also in extending the lifespan by 18 to 20 percent. I recommend a dosage of 100 mg./day.

Vitamin D is produced naturally on the skin of the body in the presence of sunlight and absorbed into the body, as we have discussed. Only if we are deprived of sunlight do we need to worry about sufficient levels of this.

Vitamin E has been mentioned in its function as an aid for heart-related problems. It has also been known, in conjunction with selenium, to slow the growth of cancer cells in blood plasma. Vitamin E is able to dissolve blood clots in the circulatory system, as well. It also improves circulation, and protects us against certain environmental toxins. By its action on free radicals, vitamin E can extend the lifespan.

The Power of Minerals

The essential difference between vitamins and minerals is that vitamins are organic (bound chemically to carbon), whereas minerals are not, except for the trace minerals selenium and chromium. Minerals necessary for good health include compounds of the basic elements calcium, chlorine, magnesium, phosphorus, potassium, and sulfur. Trace elements of the following minerals are also essential: chromium, copper, iodine, iron, manganese, molybdenum, and zinc.

Copper for Protecting Membranes and Relieving Arthritis

Copper is an important antioxidant, which inhibits free-radical formation from lack of iron, and maintains the integrity of cell membranes. It is an important defense for protecting the lung membranes of chronic smokers.

Copper bracelets have long been thought to help battle the painful symptoms of arthritis. As the copper is absorbed through sweat and skin into the body and subsequently into the synovial fluid of the affected joints, the sufferers of osteoarthritis as well as rheumatoid arthritis can expect some relief.

Magnesium for Heart and Blood Pressure

Magnesium is very important for healthy cardiac function. It is essential to the electrical and physical integrity of the heart, and also helps control blood pressure.

Manganese for Preventing Degenerative Process

Manganese, another antioxidant is so important to human biology that nature has provided for it to be substituted by magnesium in many biochemical reactions when deficiencies occur. What role does manganese play in extending your life for ten years? Well, according to the latest research, all tumors have diminished amounts of the manganese-containing enzyme. Manganese deficiency may play a role in degenerative processes in humans.

Although manganese is considered safe up to 10 mg./day, I recommend a 2 mg./day dose, since it is available in fruits, green vegetables, and whole grains, all of which I recommend highly.

Zinc for Keeping Immune System Young and Maintaining Sex Drive

Research has shown that as we age we become increasingly prone to *zinc* deficiency. Yet more than one hundred enzymes require the trace metal zinc, including the production of DNA and RNA, as well as cell membranes. Zinc is believed to maintain membrane cell integrity.

The older we get, the less efficient our immune system. If we also have less zinc in our maturing years, this may become critical. Progressive zinc deficiency may have something to do with our aging immune system. Zinc is an essential factor in this. In the laboratory, zinc-deficient animals show much greater susceptibility to cancer caused by chemicals. A certain breed of cattle (Dutch Friesian—A46 mutant) cannot absorb zinc from their feed, making them extremely susceptible to infection and early death. The cure for this terrible disease? Their lifespan is significantly increased by the mere supplementation of zinc.

For men, zinc plays an important role in sexuality. Zinc deficiency results in: lowered sex drive, regression of the testes and lower sperm count, lower testosterone levels, and lower testosterone metabolism at the cellular level. Zinc supplements may affect enlargement of the prostate, a common occurrence as men age.

There is some evidence that zinc may help those suffering from chronic rheumatoid arthritis in reducing swelling and stiffness. Since our ability to absorb zinc diminishes with age, our high-fiber diets result in lower zinc absorption, and since excessive sweating due to exercise causes a loss of existing zinc, for all these reasons, zinc supplementation is quite essential. Fortunately, most multivitamin pills contain at least 15 mg. of zinc. And I recommend 25 mg./day.

Chromium Picolinate for Reducing Cravings for Sweets and Aiding in Weight Loss

Chromium is best known for its function in supporting insulin's role in sugar metabolism. The trivalent form of chromium in the form of a substance called glucose tolerance factor is found in brewer's yeast. A deficiency in chromium results in higher cholesterol levels, cholesterol deposits in the arteries, and a shorter lifespan, as well as glucose intolerance. As we age, unfortunately, we can expect dramatic declines in the concentration of this important element in our bloodstream.

Of all the vitamins and minerals, chromium is more likely to be in short supply in the American diet than any other substance. Ninety percent of us consume less than 50 micrograms daily, even though the amount recommended by the National Academy of Science is 50 to 200 mcg. daily.

It is important to distinguish between the two types of chromium. *Trivalent* or *nutritional chromium* is the good type and has very low toxicity; *hexavalent chromium* is highly toxic, leading to skin problems and lung cancer. But there's no need to worry as far as supplements are concerned. The bad chromium would come in the form of environmental pollution. The good chromium, in the form of chromium trichloride or chromium picolinate, known as biologically active chromium, is what we find in food and supplements.

There is some intriguing evidence that chromium picolinate effectively reduces the craving for sweets and helps in losing more fat than those on similar diets without the chromium. Perhaps it is precisely because American men may be suffering from chromium deficiency that they are so susceptible to processed sweet foods.

Molybdenum for Detoxifying Harmful Substances

Molybdenum's function is to detoxify potentially harmful substances we come across daily. Although I recommend 50 micrograms per day, the amount you get in most vitamin pills (up to 25 mcg.) should be adequate. Although this substance plays an important antioxidant role, this role is very complex, and having molybdenum in the soil giving rise to the foods we eat is at least as important as its supplementary form.

Selenium for Anticancer, Antiheart Disease, Proimmune System Benefits

Finally, the superstar of trace elements: *selenium*. It used to be considered a potential carcinogen. Now it's hailed as protection *against* cancer and a number of other diseases, and as a contributor to the extension of life. Selenium serves as an antioxidant that prevents damage to cellular membranes.

Another very important aspect of selenium is its role in prevention of cancer. A growing number of studies reveals that the lower the levels of selenium in the food and water, the higher the incidence of various forms of cancer. This is true when comparing various regions of the U.S. to those of neighboring countries. Japan, for example, has a higher selenium level than the U.S. So Japanese individuals have a smaller incidence of cancer—until they emigrate to the U.S. Other research has revealed higher levels of selenium in the blood of healthy individuals than in those suffering from cancer.

Research also points to selenium as a significant boost to the immune system. Animal studies reveal that selenium supplements, when accompanied by vitamin E, lead to large increases in antibody production, as well as improved lymphocytic activity.

Selenium also acts to protect the heart and circulatory system. Research comparing different regions and countries reveals a striking relationship between selenium levels and heart disease. The lower the selenium soil content, the greater the number of deaths from heart disease. Selenium, along with vitamin E, appears to prevent free-radical damage to the blood vessels in the heart.

Selenium can act as a policing agent against other poisonous metals such as mercury and cadmium. It is hypothesized that it has this effect by combining with these metals to form inert, harmless selenides—in effect, "handcuffing" itself to these "criminal" metals to take them out of circulation.

So, for all these benefits, 200 micrograms per day is recommended. In addition to your multivitamin pill, at least consider an additional combination pill of selenium and vitamin E if you're too busy to coordinate an exact regimen.

Daily Multivitamin

A respectable multiple vitamin is the base from which to start. If nothing else, at least take this one multivitamin once a day with 500 to 1,000 mg. tablets of vitamin C as often as you need to get your optimal dosage of C. Spread the vitamin C dosage throughout the day as much as possible. Remember, this vitamin is water soluble and is not stored in the body. In addition, you might consider a B-complex tablet.

Some Cautions about Vitamins

Vitamins do not work as well in isolation as they do in concert. This is especially true of the B vitamins. So that is why a B-complex tablet is worth considering as part of your vitamin regimen.

Avoid Time-release Niacin

Vitamin B_3 (the niacin form) causes some people to feel a tingly flush over their skin. This is a normal reaction and the best way to deal with it is to see it as insurance that the vitamin is working. Niacin serves to reduce blood cholesterol levels when taken in dosages of at least 500 mg. per day. However, at levels of over 2,000 mg. a day, medical supervision should be obtained because in some very few cases temporary side effects affecting the liver have been documented. This problem has been noticed primarily with both time-release forms of niacin, and higher dosages.

Take Your Vitamins after Meals

Two cautions for vitamin C. This vitamin is somewhat acid and may cause stomach distress in high dosages in some individuals, so it is best to take this (and all other vitamins) after meals. Another way to deal with this problem if it exists is to take the vitamin in the form of *sodium ascorbate*. The second note of caution is exclusively for diabetics taking medicinal insulin. Since vitamin C increases the efficiency of insulin, it can disrupt the delicate sugar-insulin balance in diabetics. In such a case, it would be wise to have medical supervision when beginning a regimen of vitamin C.

High Blood Pressure? Consult Your Doctor

Medical supervision is also advised for those who have high blood pressure (150/90 or higher) and are taking more than 100 IU of vitamin E. Remember that this vitamin strengthens the heart muscle.

SOME CAUTIONS ABOUT MINERALS

It is important to beware of certain circumstances that would create exceptions to the rules provided for any recommended mineral regimen.

For example, anyone with preexisting high calcium concentrations in the blood should not take calcium supplementation beyond a daily multivitamin. Copper supplements should also be avoided by those suffering from hepatolenticular degeneration (Wilson's disease). Persons with renal failure should avoid magnesium beyond their daily vitamin pill as well.

Anyone with high uric acid levels or who suffers from gout should avoid molybdenum beyond their daily vitamin. Finally, selenium in dosages of 200 micrograms per day is considered to be entirely safe. But at high dosages (1,000 micrograms per day) it can become problematic. So be mindful of dosages of all your supplements, but selenium especially.

A Word of Reassurance

Having offered you cautionary advice about nutritional supplements, I now want to ease your mind that, given the conservatively moderate doses in the regimen I recommend, you are quite safe. I want to end this section on nutritional supplements with the words of Dr. Bernard Rimland, a leading theorist on nutritional therapy, who claims that, *"Vitamins are extraordinarily nontoxic.* The only vitamins that are remotely toxic are vitamins A and D, and the toxicity of vitamin A is greatly exaggerated. I think that there has been only one person in 12 years who has died of vitamin A overdose. He had to consume millions and millions of units of vitamin A."

So, as you make use of nutritional supplements to ensure the primary component of our program to add ten youthful years to your life, rest assured that what you are doing is based on years of conventional scientific research and well within the margins of safety determined by our scientific and medical communities.

SUPERFOODS FOR INCREASED BRAIN POWER

Nootropics is the name given to drugs that make the brain work better. My own research indicates that much of this lore is full of hype and exaggeration. Here is the bottom line on what works and what doesn't.

What Doesn't Work

Two of the most highly touted "smart" drugs are *deprenyl* and *piracetam*. Deprenyl, which helps the brain release the neurotransmitter dopamine, has proved successful in helping those suffering from Alzheimer's and Parkinson's diseases. By inference, it is also claimed that it might assist the normal brain in working more efficiently. But what works for the diseased brain does not necessarily help the normal brain.

Piracetam has proved successful in a few studies. In one study it is reported to have improved the alertness and aptitude of elderly drivers. In another study of only 18 elderly people, it showed "marked gains in mental performance." But much more conclusive research would be needed before I'd recommend such drugs. Let's take a look at what clearly does work.

How to B Smart

Three B vitamins—B_6, B_{12}, and folic acid—are necessary for the brain to produce the neurotransmitters *serotonin* and *norepinephrine*, which control alertness. A respectable body of evidence reveals that too little of these vitamins may result in mental sluggishness and even depression.

As we get older, we tend to produce lower levels of these vitamins. Nearly two thirds of men over 65 have low levels of at least one of these three vitamins. Among such mature individuals, those with the lowest levels of B_{12} and folic acid scored the worst on tests of memory and reasoning in a study of over 250 subjects. Correcting this deficiency proves successful in improving concentration and memory. Having adequate amounts of these B vitamins seems to part the clouds of foggy thinking.

Feeling Stressed? Can't Concentrate? Try Tyrosine!

Tyrosine is an amino acid which is converted by the brain to norepinephrine, one of the neurotransmitters mentioned previously. This substance can be depleted when we're under stress for prolonged periods. Tyrosine pills have proven effective in helping men under stress concentrate more effectively.

The Afternoon "Slump"

There are two reasons for the common afternoon slump. One has to do with time, the other with food. There seems to be a natural cycle of decreasing arousal about midafternoon affecting some individuals more than others. Some European cultures even close down their commerce for a midafternoon siesta and then open up shop again about 4 PM. We American men work right through it, or at least try to.

The other reason—food—has to do with the amount and type of food we consume for lunch. A lunch made up predominantly of carbohydrates, i.e., starchy and sweet foods, stimulates the release of insulin, which lowers the level of most amino acids but not tryptophan. The result—a drowsy, midafternoon slump. On the other hand, a lunch made up primarily of proteins causes the tryptophan to be bullied aside by the other amino acids, resulting in an alert mind able to concentrate well.

The size of the lunch matters as well. A large lunch will result in much more drowsiness than a small lunch. So the best option for an alert, effective brain and for a most productive afternoon is a rather small lunch made up of more protein than carbohydrates.

REDUCING YOUR RISK OF CANCER

The amazing thing about preventing cancer through nutrition is the simplicity of it all. Just imagine a preindustrialized farmer who has never eaten the meat of an animal or any of its products (milk, eggs); his diet is the perfect anticancer regimen.

The Low-fat, High-fiber Approach

The National Cancer Institute (NCI) recommends a lot of dietary fiber: breads made with whole grains, fruits, vegetables, and beans, as we've discussed. It urges the reduction of fat, which comes primarily from meat, fowl, and dairy products. That's exactly how our pre-industrial man eats; no sophisticated diets or supplements, are needed.

How to Eat to Prevent Cancer

But our lives aren't as simple. So here are some suggestions to begin the process of preventing the dreaded disease of cancer.

1. Help yourself to a serving of whole-grain bread, cereals, pasta, or brown rice at least four times a day. That is, have at least six servings of any of this variety of foods at least four times a day, in any combination.

2. Have at least two (1-oz.) servings each day of citrus fruits, green peppers, or tomatoes.

3. At least once a day, help yourself to some broccoli, cabbage, carrots, or cauliflower.

4. Enjoy some beans or peas a few times a week.

5. If you're not a vegetarian, choose fish or fowl (white meat) over red meat. If you must have your meat, be sure it's trimmed of fat.

What *not* to eat:

6. Avoid whole-milk dairy products such as whole milk, ice cream, and high-fat cheeses. If you must have cheese, choose 2 percent cottage or skim milk mozzarella.

7. Avoid fried foods if you know what's good for you, because butter, margarine, and shortening aren't. This includes sour cream, oil, potato chips, and so on. Air-popped popcorn is great—just say "No butter, please."

8. Never eat hot dogs, sausage, or processed luncheon meats.

Stay Within 10 Pounds of Your Ideal Weight

If you can do all this and stay within 10 pounds of your ideal weight, then you've got a good head start on keeping cancer from stealing any of those ten precious years you're earning.

The Skinny on Fat

Now for some commentary. First, on fat: As you're probably aware, there are three kinds of fat. *Saturated fats* are usually found in red meat, poultry skin, and fried foods. *Monounsaturated fats* are found primarily in peanuts and olives. *Polyunsaturated fats* are found in corn, safflower, and other cooking oils. To overcome the dietary complexity of it all, a good anticancer regimen would be to decrease saturated fats (meat and fried foods) and allow a bit more of the other two types.

How Fat Causes Cancer

It is not clear exactly how fat contributes to cancer formation. One theory holds that fat upsets the body's hormone balance and increases hormone levels of estrogen, androgen, and prolactin. Another theory maintains that bile acids, produced by the body to break down fats, create by-products which help promote the development of cancer. Whichever theory proves correct, the result is a greater vulnerability to cancer.

Whole Milk vs. Skim Milk

One notable study examined the milk-drinking habits of over 4,600 individuals. It concluded that those who drank skim milk or 2 percent milk had a significantly lower risk of cancer than those who drank whole milk. Remember that 2 percent milk has twice as much fat as skim milk, and whole milk has twice as much fat again as 2 percent milk.

But intriguingly, it was discovered that those who drank no milk at all had more cancer than those who drank skim milk. So milk is good for you (probably because of its vitamins and calcium), but only if you drink the skim variety with the lowest proportion of fat. So a very important move would be to shift from whole milk to 2 percent milk for a few weeks to get used to it. Then gradually shift to skim milk.

How Fiber Helps Prevent Cancer

One more large-scale study involving over 10,000 people revealed that diets low in fat and high in vegetables and other high-fiber foods were related to a significantly lower incidence of colon cancer. That's why I stress eating so many servings of whole-grain breads and cereals. You need to replace the fats with more fiber. The fiber not only replaces the fat; it also speeds up the movement of food in the intestines and dilutes potential carcinogens.

Peel or Wash Your Produce

Most of us are used to consuming only 10 to 12 grams of fiber a day. To help prevent cancer, we actually need about 25 to 30 grams each day. In addition to grains, don't forget fruits and vegetables—pears, apples, bananas, green beans. A wide variety works much better than focusing on any one source of fiber. This also helps prevent exposure to any one type of carcinogen that might be present as a pesticide. It also helps to wash produce well before eating or cooking. And when possible, it is advisable to peel fruits and vegetables for the same reason, even though this means losing some of the nutrients.

Why Hot Dogs Are Bad for You

One of my suggestions, earlier in this chapter, was to avoid hot dogs and sausages. Here's why: Hot dogs and most processed meats contain *sodium nitrite* and *sodium nitrate* as both a preservative and color and flavor enhancer. Nitrate by itself is harmless. But it is easily converted into nitrite, which is not. Nitrite combines with compounds called *secondary amines* to produce highly carcinogenic *nitrosamines*, either during the cooking process or during digestion. Food processors have been forced by the government to reduce nitrite levels in past years, but it is still there, albeit not as much as it used to be. So avoid hot dogs. Opt for popcorn (without butter) at baseball games.

Why Some Produce Is Waxed

Since I'm promoting fruit so highly, I need to mention this cautionary note. Many fruits and vegetables are waxed, both to prevent moisture loss and to enhance visual appeal. It is virtually impossible to know which produce have been waxed (except in such obvious cases as apples and cucumbers).

Why You Should Peel or Wash

Here's the problem. Fungicides are frequently applied before waxing, or mixed with the wax solution. Some of the FDA-approved fungicides, such as *benomyl, captan,* and *folpet* are associated with increased risk of cancer. Although this is most probably not a significant risk, because of the minute amounts per serving, it is a good idea to peel whenever possible, wash whenever you can, and, if you're able, avoid buying produce from Chile and Mexico, where higher pesticide residues are allowed.

DR. RYBACK'S ANTIAGING WEIGHT LOSS PROGRAM

There are two phases in my plan to lose weight. The first is a more or less sudden dramatic shift in your eating habits, the second a maintenance phase which ideally lasts a lifetime. There is no doubt about the importance of the first phase, as it helps establish a sense of control and mastery over your body. Most quick diets attempt this by inducing a rapid loss of water. This will result in a psychologically satisfying loss of weight in very short order. As long as weight is dramatically reduced in the short term of the beginning phase of such a diet, all appears well, on the surface.

If you are determined to experience the psychological boost, take heed: The same effect can be achieved by making a decision about some aspects of your eating habits. There is no replacement for the decrease in food intake, so one way to go about losing weight quickly is to cut your food intake drastically. Fasting is the most dramatic way to do it, but probably not the most sensible for most people. Nevertheless, some may find it effective as a starting point. So if you do consider this option, do so carefully.

How to Make Hunger Pangs Work for You

Your first concern might be that feeling of hunger that comes from the pit of your stomach. I have learned to translate that feeling as a signal that says to me that this is what it feels like to be in the process of becoming thinner. Whether you call it a process of meditation, self-hypnosis, or rationalization, the net result is that what could be considered painful and uncomfortable is suddenly transformed into a sensation of victory over obesity and mastery over one's own body. To the extent that I can really feel my hunger pangs as positive feedback to my own body, I am already being rewarded for my decrease in eating. There is no need to weigh myself in order to get this successful feedback. Eventually the "hunger pangs" become a signal for success and an instant source of self-esteem.

This process of transforming hunger pangs into positive feedback will certainly take some investment of time and energy on your part. You can begin to take 10 to 20 minutes before breakfast or before you leave home in the morning sitting in a calm, quiet spot and meditating on this process. You can either repeat to yourself silently the affirmation, "This empty sensation makes me feel thinner and successful in mastery over my own body," or merely meditate upon the process in a style that is comfortable for you.

Taking Charge

You may argue that hunger pangs are nature's way of telling you that your body needs food and that these signals should be obeyed. If you feel that way and you are as thin as you'd like to be, then you're absolutely right. However, if you are overweight, then obviously your body has been fibbing and excess weight is the unhappy result. So the choice is ultimately yours. If you are happy with your body weight, listen to the body signals to eat when you feel hunger. If, on the other hand, you want to become thinner, then you need to teach yourself to interpret your body signals in a new way. If you truly want to become thinner, then you can do so by making a conscious, intelligent decision about when you will and will not eat rather than letting your body signals make the decision for you. Having transformed your interpretation of your body signals, you are now in charge. From this vantage point, you can now decide to what degree of "suddenness" you want to become thinner.

Incidentally, one ballpark way of figuring your ideal weight is to start at 100 pounds for five feet, and then add five pounds for each additional inch, plus or minus 10 pounds.

Lose No More Than Two Pounds a Week

Eating is a very complex activity. Each culture has its own customs and traditions regarding eating. Each person also has his or her own eating habits, as well. In our culture, more specifically in the advertising aspects of our culture, we can be seduced by promises of losing 10 to 20 pounds in a single week. It is questionable whether men can actually accomplish this or not; I'd consider it quite unhealthy. A much healthier and more moderate approach, in my opinion, is to consider losing a pound or two a week at the most. Anything more sudden than that would be unproductive in the long run. Having said this, let me now offer some specific options for you to consider.

The Fasting Option

At the most extreme, you may consider the fasting option just mentioned. Fasting every other day is an option that will drastically decrease your food intake in an obvious way. Even if you eat as much food as you have always eaten on the days that you do eat, choosing this option will certainly have a dramatic impact on your weight. Some men become lightheaded and somewhat uncomfortable, even dizzy, when they try this. If you are such an individual, then this option is not for you. So let's move on to less dramatic possibilities.

The Option of Fewer Meals

The next option consists of eating only one or two meals a day rather than the usual three. If you choose this option, give considerable thought to what feels right for you. Some men feel comfortable waiting until dinner time so that they can reward themselves at the end of a day of abstinence. Others may feel they need a considerable-sized breakfast, some lunch, and then nothing for the rest of the day except for a light snack in the evening. Another option would be to have no breakfast and an early lunch or brunch, thereby condensing two meals into one.

The Most Highly Recommended Option

The healthiest option and the one I strongly recommend is to have a light breakfast, a morning snack, a light lunch, a mid-afternoon snack, and look forward to dinner as the main meal of the day. The important thing to remember here is that each time you eat, to keep it light.

BE THIN WITHOUT BEING HUNGRY

Here is a sample food plan which will keep you eating throughout the day and allow you to lose weight in the process. This is the food plan I highly recommend, in terms of minimal deprivation, nutritional sensibility, and metabolic efficiency. It's a four-step food plan that I most strongly encourage.

THE RYBACK FOOD PLAN

Breakfast
Fruit (grapefruit, orange) either whole or as juice
High-fiber cereal with skim milk, topped occasionally with fruit
Whole-wheat toast or bagel (with apple butter or jelly)

10:00 A.M.

Small apple, peach or $1/4$ cup of raisins, or English muffin

Lunch

Half cup of rice or pasta with small portions of protein such as
turkey, chicken, or seafood
Green vegetable or 1 large carrot
Mineral water, fruit juice, or skim milk
or
Bowl of your favorite homemade vegetable soup
Green salad with oil-free dressing, adorned with a small portion of
tuna, turkey breast, or sliced egg
Whole wheat roll
Fruit cup or 1 apple or 1 pear

3:00 P.M.

A fruit such as apple, peach, banana, raisins, or one cup of nonfat
yogurt

Dinner

Start with mineral water and fruit cocktail
2–3 ounces of broiled flounder, sole, skinless chicken (white meat),
or turkey breast
2 vegetables or green salad
Baked potato, pasta, or rice with Shiitake mushrooms
Whole wheat bread
Dessert of two fruits in a blender

The Ryback Food Plan allows for fruit or fruit juice 5 times a day
and allows for vegetable servings at both lunch and dinner. Whole-
wheat bread or rolls can be eaten at any of the meals. A choice of
pasta, rice, or a baked potato (without fattening condiments) is
allowed for both lunch and dinner. High-protein foods such as fish or
skinless fowl are recommended for the dinner meal, although there's
no reason not to eat such food at lunch instead if that meal is tradi-
tionally the larger one in your individual experience, or if that's your
preference for whatever reason.

I recommend you get in the habit of eating your protein food as
an "adornment" to a rice or pasta dish rather than by itself. You really don't need a lot of high-protein food, and if you get in the habit
of eating it as flavor adornment to your rice or pasta dish, you'll
enjoy it at least as much and you'll be getting into healthier eating
habits.

If you stick to the Ryback Food Plan, you won't have to worry about singling out foods that make you fat, such as fried foods, cake and cookies, candy and chocolates, creams and sauces, and high-fat dairy and beef products. Nor do you have to count calories. By flavoring your rice or pasta dishes with different high-protein foods and vegetables, you have an infinite variety of dishes you can look forward to. If you do choose to use sauces, make sure they're as fat free as possible. Rather than focus on dietary restrictions, the Ryback Food Plan focuses on what's good for you and allows you the choice to be as creative as you wish with healthy foods.

As you read through Chapter Eight on building a strong heart, you'll notice that this same food plan works for that purpose as well. The Ryback Food Plan not only keeps you thin, it will also lower your cholesterol levels and is very similar to what is recommended as a cancer-prevention diet.

For those of you who cannot bear the thought of giving up all those foods that are bad for you but seduce your taste buds, you can solve that problem by going on a food orgy one meal a week or, better yet, one meal a month. On that food "holiday" you can eat as much as you want of whatever you want, as long as you restrict it to that one time a week or month. What's really important is what happens over the long run. As long as the "orgy" meals happen only once in a while, and that helps you stay healthy the rest of the time, then that's OK. You deserve the holiday if you're eating healthy the rest of the time. This isn't about depriving you—it's about helping you live ten years longer!

SIXTEEN SIMPLE THINGS TO DO

1. Never let your clothes out to accommodate a weight gain! Instead, use the sensation of the tight-fitting clothes as a constant reminder to reduce your caloric intake. Take advantage of nature's red flag warning you of bulges and curves ahead. Then, as you lose weight, you'll be consistently rewarded on an ongoing basis as you lose pound after pound. Your clothes don't lie! Always aim to lose weight gradually. The tight-fitting clothes will act as a constant monitor, as trustworthy as any scale. Be patient in this process. You can look forward to feeling a bit more comfortable each passing week. This positive anticipation can do wonders in lifting your morale on an ongoing basis.

2. As you eat less to reduce your caloric intake, make it a habit at least to take a daily multivitamin pill. It won't add many calories (only a few, at best), but will ensure that you get the basic vitamins and minerals your body needs to stay healthy. Any good brand will do. It's best to take this pill following a meal.

3. Another component adding to your youthfulness is exercise. This need not be anything strenuous. Very moderate levels of regular activity will provide the following benefits:

   a. improved, more restful sleep;

   b. improved memory and thinking abilities;

   c. fewer psychological disturbances such as depression;

   d. less fatigue;

   e. more muscle strength and joint flexibility;

   f. more youthful heart, lungs, and cardiovascular system.

   Ponce de Leon may have gotten more benefit from his walks to and from the Fountain of Youth than from the supposed magic liquid itself. Always remember not to exert yourself initially as you begin to become active. If you're starting from a sedentary lifestyle, then walk, don't run.

   What is so important is that you start with very small steps and then very gradually increase the degree of intensity. Consistency and very gradual increases are the keys. It's taken you years to get as old as you are; give yourself some comfortable time to get younger!

4. Choose two or three of your most trusted, supportive friends and tell them you've decided to become a thinner person. Ask for their sincere support.

5. Make sure to drink six to eight glasses of water a day. The older you are, the less you can rely on your natural thirst experience to tell you how much to drink.

6. When you experience a "hunger attack," respond by doing some physical activity. Instead of going to the fridge, walk around the block, do some push-ups or sit-ups, or some stretches. You'll definitely feel better.

7. Whenever you feel hunger pangs in your stomach, let that be a signal to you that you're in the process of becoming a thinner person. Instead of letting yourself feel hungry, let yourself feel thinner. Say to yourself: "This (the hunger pang) is what it's like to be a thinner person."

8. Eat at each mealtime. The point is to eat small portions more frequently rather than large meals through the day. It's fine to allow yourself between-meal snacks if your meals and snacks are very small and made up primarily of vegetables, fruits, and grains/carbohydrates (and water).

9. Eating out creates a real dilemma. Most restaurants serve large portions, perhaps because that's what customers expect. There are two solutions: (a) Decide beforehand that you'll eat only half and take the remainder home in a "doggy bag" for another delicious meal; and (b) decide beforehand to share a meal with your partner. Ask the waiter for extra dishes. If he gives you the least bit of a hard time with that, here are some assertive options: Ask for the manager and discuss your approach to healthy eating with him (he wants happy customers), or just tell the waiter you've lost your appetite and leave. Remember that restaurants need you more than you need them.

10. If you drink alcohol, limit your intake to an ounce or two a day. Alcohol does not burn calories—it *is* calories.

11. Prepackaged foods can be deceptively high in calories. Make sure to read the ingredients carefully. Sugar is the same whether it's labeled "turbinado," "raw honey," or "fructose." Overall, it's best to minimize prepackaged, processed foods and to maximize fresh foods that you prepare yourself.

12. Except for mealtimes and planned snacks, don't make eating an activity by itself. It's easy to try to cure boredom by eating. Don't let yourself fall into this trap. Do something else if you're bored! The same thing applies to stress. Don't get into the habit of eating to deal with stress. Instead, do something physical, such as taking a brief walk, puttering in your garden, and so forth.

13. If a particularly fattening food is tempting to you, don't even bring it into your home. Remember women reciting "past the lips, onto the hips"? Well, now consider this for yourself: "Out of the store, you'll just weigh more."

14. Gradually shift from whole milk to 2 percent, to 1 percent fat milk to skim milk.

15. Avoid oat-bran muffins—if you want oats, eat it as cereal. The muffins create more problems (because of their other high-fat ingredients) than they solve.

16. Gradually diminish the amount of salad dressing you use. It's best to learn to enjoy salads without dressings at all except for such herb dressings as lemon/vinegar and powdered spices.

THE TEN COMMANDMENTS OF LOSING WEIGHT

1. Be realistic about the process of losing weight—no more than one to two pounds per week!

2. Honor and obey your commitment to your weight-loss program, no matter *what* other stresses occur in your life!

3. Do *not* allow any tempting, fattening foods into your household. Remember: "Food through the door, you'll just weigh more."

4. Do not make a habit of breaking or testing your food plan by eating a forbidden food. Remember: "Eat the wrong food, you'll look bad in the nude!"

5. *Never* rely on liquid diets to control your weight!

6. Do not eat to assuage your feelings. If you need to drown your sorrows, relieve your anxiety, cope with frustration, celebrate your joys, do *not* do it with food. Instead, do something physical or call a friend.

7. Find an exercise that is convenient and enjoyable and then, as you may have heard the familiar refrain, "Just do it!"

8. Do not try to fit exercise into your daily routine. Instead, decide on the best time for your exercise and then fit your daily routine around *it*! What's more important—that extra TV program or your health?

9. At first, learn to ignore the cues of physical hunger as well as external temptations (invitations, ads, and so on). Eat when you choose, not when the rest of the world or your stomach tells you to do so. Once you get into the habit of eating less, you and your stomach will fall into a harmonious pattern of feeling less and less hungry over time.

10. As you experience the process of becoming a thinner person, should you slip into any of the above behaviors, please be gentle with yourself, forgive yourself, and *continue in the process*.

— SIDEBAR I —

MEN'S DAILY RECOMMENDED DOSAGES OF VITAMINS

Vitamin	Approximate Daily Dosage
B_1	10 mg.
B_2	10 mg.
B_3 (niacin)	200 to 1,000 mg.
B_6	10 mg.
B_{12}	500 mcg.
Beta-carotene	25,000 IU
Biotin	300 mcg.
Choline	250 mg.
Folic Acid	400 mcg.
Inositol	500 mg.
PABA	100 mg.
Pantothenic Acid	100 mg.
C	Varies; start with 1 to 3 grams
D	400 IU
E	200 to 800 IU

— SIDEBAR II —

MEN'S DAILY RECOMMENDED DOSAGES OF MINERALS

Mineral	Approximate Daily Dosage
Calcium	1,000 mg.
Copper	3 mg.
Chromium	200 mcg.
Magnesium	400 mg.
Manganese	2 mg.
Molybdenum	50 mcg.
Selenium	200 mcg.
Zinc	25 mg.
Iodine	15 mcg.
Potassium	860 mg.

— SIDEBAR III —

HOW TO AVOID A SPARE TIRE

A spare tire is not as innocent as it may look. Studies show it may be linked to the onset of diabetes, heart disease, and high blood pressure. It may also contribute to higher cholesterol levels.

Since the tendency to develop a spare tire rises with age, it's important to know how to avoid one. Here's how to do it in 10 steps:

Smoking and Alcohol

1. Smokers are less likely to exercise vigorously and more likely to develop spare tires, so quit smoking.

2. A spare tire is also known as a beer belly. Those who have more than 2 drinks a day have a larger waist-to-hip ratio. If you do drink, limit yourself to two drinks.

Exercise

Men who don't exercise are more likely to have an "inflated" spare tire. Ongoing exercise over a six-month period will help "deflate" this tire. Here are some specific exercises:

3. Take no more than 5 minutes a day to work your abdominal muscles. Lying on your back, cross your hands over your chest, bend your knees, and lift

your shoulders 6 inches off the floor using your abdominal muscles. Hold for a few seconds before relaxing slowly back to the floor. Do as many slow repetitions as you can in a 5-minute period.

4. As you diet, lean muscle tissue is lost along with fatty tissue, so it's important to keep building your muscles. The more muscle you build and maintain, the higher your metabolism, and the more weight you'll end up losing. An extra 2 pounds of muscle can be expected to burn off 200 more calories a day. The best way to build muscle is through weight lifting. Here are some suggestions:

   a. To build upper body musculature, get a rowing machine or use the one at your local Y or health spa.

   b. While there, ask the instructor to show you how to use free weights and universal machines.

   c. To build hip and leg muscles, become familiar with stairmasters, treadmills, and stationary bikes.

5. Make it a point to take a leisurely stroll for about 3 miles daily. Doing it at the same time each day will make it easier to be consistent. Do some form of exercise at least four times a week; consistency is the key to your avoiding that spare tire.

Diet

6. In this chapter, weight loss has been discussed at length. Slow, consistent food control is what will keep that spare tire from inflating. Dramatic diets will contribute to your spare tire. Plus, remember to keep your food intake under control. Comfortable and consistent does it best.

7. In order to keep your metabolism from slowing down and helping to inflate your spare tire, rather than cutting your food intake drastically, stick to the Ryback Food Plan and eat five times a day. This keeps the insulin stabilized at a lower level in your body. Less fat will be stored if you can keep the insulin level down.

8. For similar reasons, avoid simple sugars found in soft drinks and candy. These sugars promote the release of insulin, which in turn, "opens up" the fat cells to absorb whatever fat is in the bloodstream. Most important, never eat simple sugars along with fat in the same meal.

Stress Reduction

9. Research has shown that stress increases the level of cortisol in the body, and this seems to correlate with more distribution of fat to the abdomen. Stress leads to adrenaline output, which causes a release of fat from fat cells all over the body. Cortisol then takes the unused fat and tends to favor

the mid-section when it's redeposited. So cutting down on stress will help keep your spare tire from inflating.

10. If you can't reduce the stress factors impinging on your life, then at least take 10 minutes a day and learn to do simple meditation. Some time before breakfast or dinner, find a quiet place, free from distraction, and sit quietly, eyes closed, while thinking "one" as you breathe in and "two" as you breathe out. As you continue, breathe slowly and relax your muscles. If thoughts intrude, welcome them and then let them go their way as you mentally wave good-bye to them. With time, the intruding thoughts will decrease in frequency and you'll find yourself in a totally relaxed frame of mind.

— SIDEBAR IV —

FOODS HIGH IN FIBER
(in descending order)

Fruit
Raspberries
Pears
Raisins
Prunes

Vegetables
Kidney beans
Peas
Potato
Broccoli

Grains
100% bran cereal
Oat bran
Corn Bran
Whole-wheat bread

— SIDEBAR V —

CAROTENE: FRIEND OR ENEMY?

Over 100 studies over the past 15 years have pointed to beta-carotene as an antioxidant which helps to prevent cancer. One large-scale study, however, has implicated beta-carotene as possibly *increasing* the likelihood of cancer.

Beta-carotene is only one of a great many carotenoids but is best-known because it's the best vitamin-A precursor and because it's so plentiful. Research has borne out that those who eat the most vegetables high in beta-carotene have the *lowest levels of cancers of the lung, stomach, cervix, prostate, and colon.* Alternately, it was found that those eating the least beta-carotene-rich foods had *7 times* the lung cancer risk of those who ate the most.

The recent Finnish study of over 29,000 smokers, however, found higher levels of lung cancer among those taking beta-carotene pills, as well as an 8 percent higher death rate over all. How come?

Here are some possible answers:

1. Many of the smokers may have entered the study with pre-existing tumors.

2. There was a high number of dropouts in the study, skewing the outcome unfavorably.

3. The results were significant at the .01 level of probability. What this means is that there's a 1 in 100 chance that the results are not correct.

4. There may be an essential difference between manufactured pills (used in the study) and beta-carotene in its natural form in foods. Most pills contain only one of a variety of forms of the beta-carotene found naturally in foods.

5. Even if the results are "true," they may not be "true" for healthy people who *don't* smoke.

Overall, the ongoing research points to beta-carotene, even in supplement form, as promoting longer life. But your best bet is to make sure to include *foods* high in beta-carotene in your diet. Make sure to include a daily intake of at least one serving of carrots, cantaloupe, or sweet potato in your diet. It may help add years to your life.

— SIDEBAR VI —

No-Pain Grains

Grain (1 cup)	Water (cups)	Simmer for	Let Stand	Yield (cups)
Amaranth	3	25 min.	0 min.	2
Barley (pearled)	3	50 min.	10 min.	$3^1/_2$
Brown rice	$2^1/_2$	45 min.	10 min.	$3^1/_2$
Buckwheat groats	2	12 min.	5 min.	2
Bulgur	2	15 min.	5 min.	3
Couscous	2	0 min.*	10 min.	3
Millet	2	25 min.	5 min.	$3^1/_2$
Quinoa	2	15 min.	5 min.	3
Triticale**	$2^1/_4$	$1^3/_4$ hr.	10 min.	2
Wheat berries**	$3^1/_2$	1 hr.	15 min.	2
Wild rice	$2^1/_4$	45 min.	10 min.	$2^1/_2$

Instructions:

1. Boil the water and add the grain.
2. Bring the water back to a boil, cover, and reduce the heat to a simmer.
3. After simmering, remove the pot from the burner and let stand, covered.

   * Put the couscous into a bowl, add the boiling water, cover and let stand.
   ** Soak overnight before cooking.

Chart adapted from *Recipes from an Ecological Kitchen,* by Lorna J. Sass (William Morrow and Co., 1992).

— SIDEBAR VII —

Foods High in Beta-Carotene

Apricots	Spinach
Broccoli	Squash
Carrots	Sweet Potatoes

— SIDEBAR VIII —

Foods High in Calcium

Food	Milligrams of Calcium
1 cup of nonfat yogurt	300
3 oz. sardines	320
1 cup skim milk	300
3 oz. salmon	180
3 oz. tofu	175
1/2 cup collard greens	150
1/2 cup cooked spinach	120
1/2 cup boiled broccoli	90
1/2 cup white beans	80

— SIDEBAR IX —

Ideal Weight for Men

Height		Frame		
Ft	In	Small	Medium	Large
5	2	128–134	131–141	138–150
5	3	130–136	133–143	140–153
5	4	132–138	135–145	142–156
5	5	134–140	137–148	144–160
5	6	136–142	139–151	146–164
5	7	138–145	142–154	149–168
5	8	140–148	145–157	152–172
5	9	142–151	148–160	155–176
5	10	144–154	151–163	158–180
5	11	146–157	154–166	161–184
6	0	149–160	157–170	164–188
6	1	152–164	160–174	168–192
6	2	155–168	164–178	172–197
6	3	158–172	167–182	176–202
6	4	162–176	171–187	181–207

Based on a weight-height mortality study conducted by the Society of Actuaries and the Association of Life Insurance Medical Directors of America. *Metropolitan Life Insurance Company, revised 1983.*

Height includes 1-in. heel. Weight includes 5 pounds for indoor clothing.

— CHART I —

Vitamin	Functions
A	Purifies the blood from pollutants. Essential to night vision and tissue growth. Retards development of cancerous tumors.
Thiamine	Vital to energy metabolism.
Riboflavin	Important to energy metabolism.
B_3 (Niacin)	Reduces cholesterol.
B_6	Protects against cancer. Helps keep skin healthy. Boosts immune system.
Pantothenic Acid	Relieves painful symptoms of rheumatoid arthritis.
Folate (Folic Acid)	Important for growth and healthy blood.
B_{12}	Helps process of blood clotting. Important in growth and metabolism.
C	Firms capillary walls. Important in formation of collagen. Helps regulate normal cholesterol levels.
D	Regulates bone growth.
E	Aids in heart-related problems. Improves circulation. Helps dissolve blood clots in circulatory system.
K	Essential for formation of protein in the body.

— CHART II —

Minerals	Functions
Calcium	Aids in bone growth.
Chromium picolinate	Supports insulin's role in sugar metabolism. Helps regulate cholesterol levels. Reduces craving for sweets.
Copper	Maintains integrity of cell membranes.
Magnesium	Essential to electrical and physical integrity of heart.

Manganese	Antioxidant. Deficiency leads to degenerative process.
Molybdenum	Detoxifies harmful substances.
Selenium	Helps protect against cancer. Helps prevent damage to cellular membranes.
Zinc	Essential to many human enzymes. Keeps immune system young.

EXERCISE
AWAY THE YEARS

According to the American Heart Association, lack of exercise is one of 11 factors that predispose us to heart disease. And as for our concern about "creeping" overweight, I'm convinced that inactivity is as important a factor as overeating. Unequivocally, exercise slows the aging process. So for a healthier heart, a slimmer body, and a longer life, try getting off your duff for starters.

I know, you have a good number of convincing reasons not to. You don't have time. You're overstressed with time demands as it is. Why add to the stress by putting more time demands on your life? For there's no getting around the fact that exercise takes time; we even measure it in units of time (a 45-minute workout, 30-minute jog, and so on).

Besides that, exercise is painful and sweaty—how can that be any fun! "Sure," you'd like me to reassure you, "sit back and relax! Life is too short!"

"Made shorter," you won't want me to add, "by the greater inevitability of obesity, coronary disease, high blood pressure and its companion in old age, stroke, and a generally sickly disposition."

Have I talked you into some movement yet? Well, consider this: Heart attacks are the leading cause of death in both men and women. One out of five men, by the time they reach 60, will have had a heart attack.

HOW EXERCISE PROLONGS YOUR LIFE

1. Decreases your risk of heart attack.

2. Aids your heart in doing its job more effectively.

3. Helps your body use oxygen more effectively.

4. Improves circulation throughout your body.

5. Lowers blood pressure.

6. Lowers cholesterol.

7. Helps you lose weight more effectively by burning fat and raising your metabolism.

8. Makes your muscles both stronger and more elastic.

9. Enhances your immune system (except for a few hours after grueling marathons).

10. Decreases stress and the destructive effects of depression.

Even 14 Minutes a Day Will Make a Difference

Over 16,000 men between the ages of 40 and 64 were studied by the British scientist, J. N. Morris, who compared those who included at least 14 uninterrupted minutes a day of running, swimming, or bicycling in their ongoing lifestyle with those who were inactive. Those who reported such regular, vigorous exercise in their lives suffered only one-third the number of heart attacks as did their less active counterparts. So you see, it doesn't take much activity to result in a very important health difference.

In a more thorough investigation of over 500 of these same men, electrocardiogram data indicated that the inactive men showed twice as many heart abnormalities as did the exercising group.

Active Work Means Fewer Fatal Heart Attacks

Here in America, a long-term study of over 20 years on more than 6,000 San Francisco Bay longshoremen (a study not to be taken lightheartedly) revealed, when all the data were scientifically sorted out to allow for individual differences, that high energy output on the job substantially reduced the risk of fatal heart attack. Less active workers were three times more likely to die of a heart attack than their more active counterparts.

The data also revealed that those who were less active, smoked heavily, and had high blood pressure were *twenty* times as likely to suffer a fatal heart attack as their counterparts who had none of these three characteristics.

How to Be Completely Immune to Heart Disease

At least one scientist believes that it is possible to become entirely immune to heart disease, by increasing the level of activity to a certain criterion. And just what is that specific criterion? According to Dr. Tom Bassler, it is the ability to complete a marathon. Beginning in 1967, Dr. Bassler did an ongoing, worldwide analysis of the deaths of marathon runners. After histological analysis of over 200 such deaths, not one proved to be from heart disease. Responding to challenges from the medical community, Dr. Bassler does submit that such immunity lasts only while the runner is in training.

Scientific Proof That Exercise Lengthens the Lifespan

What about proof of the effect of exercise to prolong life? Such data is more attainable from animal research than human research, for reasons that begin to become obvious once you think about it. It is much easier to do lifespan research on animals because the researcher is more likely to outlive his subjects. In addition, it would be unethical to manipulate factors in human lives that might end up shortening them. So we're more likely to rely on rodents rather than humans for such research. I'll mention only two such studies.

With mice allowed to engage in wheel exercise, it has been found that males were able to extend their lifespan by 10 percent. Perhaps the exercise didn't start early enough; the mice were almost two years old at the beginning of the study.

A more long-term study, in which rats began 10-minute exercise sessions on a motor-driven drum at one month of age (about three years old in human terms), was conducted by Ohio State University. In this lifelong study, the lifespan of the exercising rats was 31 percent longer than their relatively less active counterparts. This time both males and females were equally affected.

So this research implies that if we start real early, exercise can lengthen our lifespans considerably. But even if we begin at the age of senior citizens, we can still aspire to an added few years of productive life.

Exercise and Moderate Food Intake

Losing weight through a combination of reduced food consumption *and* exercise is superior to losing weight through food reduction alone. With exercise, more body fat is lost with virtually no loss in muscle tissue.

DR. RYBACK'S SPEAR METHOD FOR GETTING STARTED

If you happen to be a sedentary type, it is extremely important that you have a medical checkup as well as a fitness evaluation prior to starting your exercise regimen. Your doctor will most likely take a medical history, including questions about illness in your family, and perform a physical exam, including a blood analysis and an electro-cardiogram. If you're over 40, an exercise treadmill study or stress test will pick up any apparent problems with your heart.

For getting started (or restarted), allow me to share an acronym I've used for myself: SPEAR.

S—Set a goal: losing five pounds, fitting into your tight clothes, winning a trophy, running a marathon.

P—Pick an exercise you like, one that is compatible with your schedule, that fits in logistically with your life (near a park, pool, airport, and so on).

E—Enjoy. Not only should you enjoy the activity itself, but allow music, the right companion(s), and sense of competition to fulfill their roles. When running, I enjoy anticipating the Saturday morning road races. When swimming, I enjoy the feminine pulchritude adorning the pool. To each his own—find your own.

A—Always do your exercise. Make it a high priority in your daily schedule. Don't allow exceptions to become the rule. I discipline myself by not having my dinner until I've done my run or swim. I usually end up running when I get hungry enough.

R—Routine is extremely helpful. If I'm running, I make sure my running gear is handy and my Walkman batteries are recharged, so when the time comes, I won't have to mess with those things and become distracted. Same with swimming. Do I have my goggles and dry swimsuit handy when the time comes? If you can do your activity the same time each day, all the better. The more routine the logistics, the easier you'll make it for yourself.

CREATE YOUR OWN FITNESS PLAN

Ted is a 48-year-old businessman who continually complains about aches and pains. He works hard, long hours and plays an intense game of basketball once a week. During the week there are practice sessions for the team, but Ted is usually too busy to attend.

Ted first came to my office to figure out ways to reduce the stress in his life. His business was going through rough times. His wife had been helping him in his business but she had left him and so he had the double trouble of losing his marriage and his "business partner."

In addition to discussing his relationship with his wife and ways of reducing stress (see Chapter 3), we also discussed which activities would be most suitable for his situation. There are a whole host of possibilities available for men of different builds and different ages. I went over some of these with Ted.

The most popular aerobic activities are jogging, walking, and swimming. But any activity that has you moving, whether it's competitive sports or domestic activities such as gardening or housecleaning, or even sex, will do you more good than remaining a sedentary couch potato.

Here is a partial list of sports and activities from which you can choose to create your own fitness plan.

1. Jogging or Running (the speed is the difference)

For many years, this has been the most popular choice, resulting in mammoth events, such as the Bay to Breakers Run in San Francisco, the Peachtree Road Race in Atlanta, and the Boston Marathon.

This activity can be highly enjoyable alone, in small groups, or in large social events, and provides the benefits of a stronger cardiovascular system, a leaner body, and stronger legs.

One downside of running is that some men may experience wear and tear on their joints, resulting in some aches and pains around the ankles, knees, or hips, especially as the years go by.

Another downside is the dependency on the vagaries of weather. But this can easily be overcome by jogging on indoor tracks during inclement weather.

2. Swimming

Swimming is much more of a solo activity, except for sharing the body of water with others. Since indoor pools are often available, the weather is less of a problem here. Also, you may get a chance to observe the latest in swimsuit fashions to brighten your daily exercise.

Swimming is a great all-round shaper of muscles. Whatever stroke you choose, you're likely to use almost all your long muscles, both upper and lower body. You may lose weight a bit more slowly than in running because you'll tend to build more muscle swimming. But your overall shape will definitely improve. Also, your joints will not be subjected to the strains that most other physical activities involve.

3. Cycling

Cycling enables you to enjoy the outdoors to your heart's delight. You can cycle around your neighborhood or take trips with groups that turn into highly enjoyable social events. You can cycle at your leisure or compete with svelte men and women in local and national competitions. Your joints don't take much of a beating unless you slip and fall. So wear good protection, especially an effective helmet.

Cycling works virtually all muscles of the body, but especially the legs, of course. The downsides: dependence on the weather and the dangers of traffic.

4. Weight Training

It's quite evident that this activity is more of a muscle builder than a cardiovascular challenge, although many repetitions (reps) with smaller weights can be designed for cardiovascular fitness as well. There are so many possibilities here in terms of choosing which muscles to build and to what extent and how (bigger and more prominent or more svelte and compact). The two main categories into which this activity falls are *free weights* (hand weights and barbells) and machine training (Nautilus and universal machines, and multistation gyms).

In a recent YMCA study, it was shown that some individuals could gain up to 6 pounds of muscle and lose up to 15 pounds of fat in just seven weeks of tri-weekly 20-minute sessions. Their svelte, muscular bodies probably looked a few years younger too. So if looking ten years younger is one of your goals, this activity should be high on your list along with my antiaging food plan.

Weight-training technology has really blossomed in the recent past, and so it's a good idea to consult with a trainer at your local gym as you start out. Doing the wrong thing in the beginning (starting with weights that are too heavy, performing too many reps, or following the wrong sequence or combination of exercises) can really put a dent in your workout. Seek a trainer's advice.

The best thing about this activity is that you can focus directly on the area of your body that you want to work on. Each muscle group has its own set of exercises designed to build its strength. You can literally sculpt your own body, if you're willing to put in the time and effort. That's how Arnold Schwarzenegger, once a skinny Austrian teenager, started out.

5. Tennis

Tennis is a great way to get physical if you're bored by most other activities but you enjoy socializing. You can make new friends, look your manliest in tennis shorts, and enjoy keen competition in singles and doubles matches. (Don't forget mixed doubles for those more socially inclined.)

If you're new to this game, you'll do well to take lessons at first and then work your way toward higher skill levels in the league you join.

6. Basketball

Basketball is more appropriate for those men with lots of energy and limber joints. A false step can involve a sprained ankle or worse, so you be the judge of your own suppleness. But an easy game of one-on-one or two-on-two can be managed by practically all body types.

7. Soccer

This sport involves much vigor and stamina—great for wind and strong legs. It's a fairly demanding sport but one that is filled with the strong cooperative spirit of your teammates. Having a relaxing drink after the game contributes to this sense of camaraderie.

8. Badminton

Skill-intensive a sport as any, this will get you sweating out your workaday tensions and provide opportunity for social networking—with business associates, the opposite sex, or even business associates of the opposite sex.

9. Volleyball

Another active sport, for novices as well as veterans, volleyball is a sport that offers a workout without too much strain and an opportunity for casual socializing. A fairly laid-back activity which can occasionally be hot and heavy, this is a good selection for those who have problems with commitment, as well as for those who want an ongoing serious involvement.

10. Golf

Talk about a relaxed sport! Just walk along (leaving the cart behind) and hit that little ball with a stick. Oh, but doesn't it take a lifetime of learning that skill to do it well! And here's a sport you can do the rest of your life and keep getting better at it.

11. Walking

Alone or with your buddies, in silence or with earphones, indoor or outdoor, relaxed or brisk, walking is a very versatile activity you can do anytime, and practically anywhere.

12. Stairclimbing

Not necessarily on machines, this can be done wherever there are stairs—at home or at work. Great for your leg muscles and buttocks.

13. Aerobics

This can be done at home to videos or at the gym in group formation. Either way, it can be lots of fun, especially in co-ed groups. A good instructor will target muscle groups all over your body. Videos can be selected with different focal interests.

14. Yardwork

Mowing, raking, weeding, and planting can really challenge your body if you do it in earnest for an hour or longer. It's slow exercise that you can do at your leisure, and then take pride in the results of your efforts.

15. Sex

Although this requires a partner to be done well, I categorize it as an individual activity since, in most cases, the two of you will be doing it in privacy. Sex is one way to get a good workout for your whole body without even giving that aspect of the experience a second thought. Do what comes naturally, let it last a while, and your muscles are bound to get a decent workout. Fun, too, according to the latest research.

CUSTOMIZE YOUR WORKOUT

When it comes to workouts, never has the phrase "different strokes for different folks" been more apt. Depending on your age, weight, energy level, schedule, and budget, you may choose one activity over another. To assist you in this decision-making process, here's a chart with some suggestions.

Based on your age, energy level, and body type, this chart suggests the activities you might choose as starting points. As you progress, be flexible in trying new activities as your schedule and budget allow, and as your interests guide you.

Here are some guidelines, according to your body type:

Ectomorphs

If you've got a tendency to remain thin, you're probably high in energy with above-average endurance. Chances are you eat more than most, yet remain quite slim.

Since you tend to be light in muscle as well as fat, I recommend weight training for all age levels and all energy levels. Since your light weight makes you vulnerable to injury in team sports, I recommend that only for those men with higher energy levels.

Since I recommend weight training for ectomorphs at all ages and energy levels, I want to share some general guidelines to help you get started. I'll assume you want to build muscle definition rather quickly so you can see some visible results from all your efforts.

1. Focus on your exercise program, not on socializing. It's tempting to "hang out" and banter with other guys about what you're doing to build your physique. Your time is limited. Do what you've come to do and get the job done. It takes a lot of repetitions (reps) to get those muscles bulging.

2. Be sure to drink your 8 glasses of water daily. You'll need this especially as your muscles grow.

3. Warm up with each exercise by going through the motions with a very light weight. Then immediately go to the heaviest weight of which you're capable and fatigue your muscles by doing as many reps as you can. For your second set, decrease the weights by 5 to 15 pounds or whatever weight it takes for you to complete 8 to 10 reps before your muscles are fatigued. Keep experimenting along these lines till you're selecting the right weights for this "count-down" procedure. Then just watch your muscles grow.

4. Slow down and count to 10. As you lift each weight, do it slowly to a count of 10. Then as you lower it, do so to a count of 4. This will engage more muscle fibers for longer time periods, resulting in bigger muscles acquired more quickly. This is clearly a case of getting there more quickly by moving more slowly.

Mesomorphs

If you have a good set of muscles without much fat on a medium build, running, team sports, and cycling are good activities for most of you. The loss in weight you might achieve through running and cycling won't hurt you. Your well-centered body type makes team sports a good choice for those of you who are more energetic.

Endomorphs

With a tendency to put on weight, swimming is a great start for you, first, because your body type will give you buoyancy in the water, and second, because you need the intensity of swimming exercise to transform some of that fat into shapely muscle.

I don't recommend running as a starting point for you because the extra weight may damage your knees or other joints.

AGE	Ectomorph			Mesomorph			Endomorph		
over 20	WT	WC	IW	RT	RT	IC	SW	ST	IC
over 40	WT	WC	IW	TC	TC	IC	SW	SC	IS
over 60	SW	SW	SW	SW	SW	SW	SW	SW	IW
Energy level	high	med	low	high	med	low	high	med	low

KEY:

C = Cycling
I = Individual activities
R = Running
S = Swimming
T = Team sport
W = Weight lifting

BE YOUR OWN PERSONAL TRAINER:
SIX TIPS FOR STICKING TO A WORKOUT PROGRAM

1. Begin Slowly and Build Gradually

If you start with walking or jogging, use your THR to guide you. Whatever you do, it's terribly important that you begin very slowly and increase your intensity very gradually. The worst thing you can do is try too hard initially and burn yourself out before allowing your form of exercise to become a habit.

2. Walk with Friends or Music

If you're walking, explore different routes if you can. Do all you can to make the walk enjoyable. A Walkman with your favorite music or an interesting and equally devoted companion will do wonders to make this activity enjoyable. And it must be enjoyable if it's going to last.

3. Run for the Glory

Music or a companion will also help jogging. As you slowly gain your distance, you can begin exploring the possibility of joining the many Saturday morning friendly walks and runs that offer small trophies and T-shirts if you compete successfully in your age group.

4. How to Deal with Bad Weather

If you're a walker and you don't live in a safe area or you don't like bad weather (hot or cold), you can drive to your city airport (or mall) and walk indoors.

5. The Secret to Successful Exercising

Whatever your choice, try to do it the same time every day. Otherwise, everything else will take priority and your exercise will fall through the cracks. Some men enjoy getting up earlier than usual and completing their exercise to start their day. Others will use their lunch time and reward themselves with a light lunch (yogurt and fruit, for example) and have an alert, productive afternoon while their well-fed colleagues struggle to stay awake on a full belly and martini. Still other men prefer to wait until the end of the day and use their exercise to unwind from the stresses of the day. Whatever time you choose, make it a consistent routine, so that there's no decision to make at the time. In my opinion, that's the secret to successful aerobic exercising.

6. Use the Best Accessories

As for equipment, this is one aspect of your life in which you need to be good to yourself. Get the best walking or running shoes you can afford. And get good advice from a knowledgeable salesperson at the time of purchase. For swimming, all you need is a good pair of swim goggles and probably a rubber swim cap. And of course a swimsuit, unless you have a private pool.

SIX BACK-STRENGTHENING EXERCISES

If you want to strengthen your back, make a commitment to 15 minutes a day during which you can do each of the following exercises five times. Do this 3 to 5 days a week. If you have a bad back, check with your doctor first.

1. Lie on your stomach with elbows bent by your sides and hands flat on the floor. Keeping your hips on the floor, slowly lift your upper body until you feel a slight stretch in your lower back. Hold for 15 seconds.

2. In the same position, place a small pillow under your stomach. With your arms held against your sides, raise your head and shoulders just off the floor. Count to 5, then gradually lower yourself.

3. In the same position, keeping arms extended straight above your head, raise your right arm and left leg and hold for a count of 5. Then repeat with your left arm and right leg.

4. Turn over on your back, placing the pillow under the small of your back, and bend one knee while keeping the other flat on the floor. Grab the bent leg just behind the knee and pull gently toward your chest until you feel the pull in your lower back. Repeat for the other leg.

5. Repeat this with both legs, rolling your shoulders forward, tucking your chin to your chest and lifting your shoulders a few inches off the floor.

6. In the same position, bend both knees with your feet flat on the floor, and your arms, palms down, along your sides. Lift your head and shoulders gently off the floor and hold for a count of five. Return and rest for at least 10 seconds before repeating.

EXERCISE FOR BETTER SEX

We get better with practice, and that goes for sexual endurance as it does for anything else. Men usually (but not always) are the more active in sexual positioning and movement. So here are some exercises that will put you in excellent form for better sex.

Working from top down, muscles important to sexual fitness are the shoulders (the better to hold you, my dear), abdominals (for better thrust), hips and groin (where the action is).

Shoulders

The trick is not only strength for the shoulders, which you get from lifting weights and other upper-body exercise—but also flexibility. Rolling around in the hay requires flexibility under, around, and on top of the shoulders.

For best results, straighten your arms in front of you, grab your left wrist with your right hand and extend your arms up above your head and slightly backward until you feel the gentle pull under your armpits. Hold for a count of 5, then relax your arms, and repeat once or twice.

Abdominals

Perhaps the most important muscles for a man's lovemaking, the abdominals can be strengthened by well-known curls. Lying on your back with knees bent, and arms folded across your chest or clasped behind your neck for support, slowly bring your head and shoulders up until your shoulders are 4 inches off the floor. Hold for a count of 3, then relax and repeat, as often as you feel comfortable. Slowly increase the number as you get familiar with this exercise.

Hips and Groin

Flexibility is the key here rather than strength, and two exercises can help you attain this. Here's the first. Seated on the floor with your legs together and bent knees apart, reach for your ankles with your elbows between your knees. Now grasp your ankles and allow your soles to come together against one another. Bend forward slightly as you allow the pressure of your elbows against your knees to force your knees down toward the floor ever so gently. When you feel the pull in your groin, stop and hold for a few seconds. Relax your hold and repeat two or three times, making sure to be very gentle.

For the second exercise, sit with your legs crossed and lean forward slightly with your arms stretched out in front of you. When you feel the pull in your groin, lean into it very gently once or twice more. Relax and repeat 2 or 3 times.

Kegel Exercises

First discovered in the '40s by Dr. Arnold Kegel in order to help women gain better bladder control, these exercises can also help men attain firmer erections, have more intense orgasms more often, and enjoy greater staying power.

The muscles in focus here are those that control the flow of urine. There are three basic exercises, and all are fairly simple to describe, if not to carry out. For the first, imagine your intention to stop the flow of urine once it has begun. You can feel the muscle deep within your groin tense up. Do this and hold for a count of three.

For the second exercise, clench and relax these same muscles as quickly as you can.

For the third exercise, imagine forcing out the last drops of urine after voiding your bladder. This time you'll feel your abdominal walls tighten up as well.

Complete 10 slow reps of each of these exercises about 5 times a day. After a while, you'll feel more sensitive and in control of your orgasms. Some men can also attain longer-lasting orgasms once they become proficient in these exercises.

You've now got all the expertise to tune your body muscles to become a great lover. The rest is up to you.

PUSHING 90, PUMPING IRON

Weight lifting prolongs life by slowing down or eliminating the effects of arthritis, lung disease, and other conditions, even for 90-year-olds. A recent study of 50 frail, elderly nursing home residents, average age, 87, some well over age 90, the eldest being 98, surveyed the effects of hip and knee resistance exercises. The result of 10 weeks of these exercise regimens three times a week was greater strength and muscle size as well as improved mobility and more spontaneous activity.

Sol, for instance, at 91 years of age was limited to shuffling along slowly to keep up with his younger wife Celia, a sprightly 82 years of age. A lack of exercise kept Sol looking and feeling disabled. Once he began a comfortable regimen of easy leg exercises, he felt more comfortable climbing stairs without assistance and keeping up with his youthful wife. Enjoying their golden years together, Sol and Celia can now be seen together during their daily sojourns, arm in arm, enjoying the afternoon sun. Pushing 92, Sol is now able to enjoy his youthful wife even more fully.

Here are the 10 Commandments of staying fit forever, at least until you finish enjoying those ten extra years of good health in an attractive body.

STAYING FIT FOREVER

1. Find an exercise activity you enjoy.
2. Find friends to join you.
3. Begin slowly, build gradually.
4. If possible, do it to music you enjoy.

5. Do it the same time each day.

6. Do a minimum of 30 to 45 minutes three times a week.

7. Vary your workout.

8. Eat less.

9. Share your new fitness with your lover in sexy ways.

10. Don't slack off as the years go by.

Only by continuing to stay active through the passing years, with physical activities that you really enjoy, will you be able to count on adding healthy years to your life through exercise. Success begets success, and physical activity begets fitness. The worst thing you can do to your body is to allow it to lay fallow. Stay active and you'll live longer. Stay true to a challenging regimen of enjoyable exercise and just watch your mirror to witness measurable changes that will inspire you.

— SIDEBAR I —

DETERMINING YOUR TARGET HEART RATE

Aerobic exercise, done for at least 30 minutes, stimulates the entire body and reaches maximum effect as you reach your Target Heart Rate (THR). This often appears to be a complicated procedure to figure out numerically, so let's take a few minutes now to master that and get it out of the way.

First, start with the number 220, then subtract your age. Now from that figure subtract your resting heart rate (usually between 60 and 80). Since you're a beginner, multiply the new number by 60 percent. To that, add your resting heart rate. The number you now have is your THR. Divide by 6, so that you can take your pulse for 10 seconds to see if you've reached your THR.

It's worthwhile going through a theoretical example to make sure you've got it right. Once you have it, you can use it for a long time. Let's assume you're 40 and that your resting heart rate is 70.

Step 1   220 – 40 (age) = 180

Step 2   180 – 70 (resting heart rate) = 110

Step 3   110 × 60% (for beginners) = 66

Step 4   66 + 70 (resting heart rate) = 136

Step 5   136 : 6 (ten-sec. interval) = 22 or 23

Now when you exercise, you can take your pulse for 10 seconds to see how close you've come to your THR. Your THR is your ideal goal. If you're below it, you can push yourself harder. If you're above, slow down for awhile.

— SIDEBAR II —

THE TV WORKOUT

The 3 Reasons We Eat While Watching TV

There may be a psychological reason to explain the fact that so many people eat while watching television. Here's what I think:

1. My feeling is that while sitting still for extended hours, the body has a tendency to want to be active. Since we don't move around much while watching TV, one of the "activities" we engage in is eating.

2. A second reason may be that watching TV is, more than being passive, a receptive modality. That is, we are "taking in" the entertainment before us. Consequently, "taking in" food is in the same modality, and therefore the temptation to eat is very seductive at that time. (The same reasoning applies to eating snacks during movies. Movie theaters make as much, if not more, on popcorn, candy, and soft drinks as they do on the tickets themselves.)

3. A third reason has to do with the preponderance of TV commercials on food products.

All these serve to make us very susceptible to accompanying our TV watching with eating behaviors. Even now, I still find it hard to resist these temptations while watching TV.

One solution that has worked very well for me is to arrange my living room in such a way that I have some exercise apparatus next to the sofa in front of the TV so that I can easily move to that apparatus and become active on it instead of filling my mouth with food. For me, it really feels as if the exercise is an effective substitute for the activity of eating. As a matter of fact, it would be ideal to have a few exercise options to provide a variety instead of the potential of boredom with a single exercise. For example, it would be great to have an exercycle, a rowing machine, and some barbells. That way, you could switch from one to the other as you liked. This has the obvious advantage of not only avoiding too much snacking, but also getting your body fit at the same time.

KEEPING
YOUR HEART STRONG

As we age, we become susceptible to a nasty substance that collects on the inner walls of our arteries. As these initial deposits of fat and debris accumulate, they begin to protrude into the inner surface of the blood vessels. Eventually, blockage of certain arteries becomes a danger.

WHAT CAUSES HEART ATTACKS

This process may occur anywhere in the body, but is particularly dangerous when it occurs in the arteries that feed the heart itself. Two dangerous possibilities may occur. If an artery to the heart is completely occluded, starving some heart tissue of oxygen and causing the death of that tissue, we have a heart attack.

The other possibility is that the occlusion is not great enough to stop the blood flow by itself, but is sufficiently narrow that the blood cells passing through it may begin to stick together in the narrow passage, forming a clot, and the occlusion becomes complete, starving and killing heart tissue as before.

Either of these events may cause a sharp, but temporary pain which we may choose to dismiss as heartburn, for that is what it might very well feel like. The heart, in most cases, continues to function, but with a bit of a handicap.

The Purpose of Cholesterol

Fat is not the same as cholesterol. Some fat is obviously needed by the body. Fat will not mix with the blood in the body (oil and water don't mix; nor do fat and blood), so a messenger or transport device is necessary. That's where cholesterol comes in. A certain amount of cholesterol is actually vital to life itself. It is manufactured by our livers, but we can also get it from animal foods we eat, such as meat and eggs.

Good Cholesterol vs. Bad Cholesterol

When we eat fat, it is digested and goes first to the liver, where it is combined with cholesterol to be sent to other parts of the body. There are basically two types of cholesterol in one's system, which we can, for simplicity, refer to as bad cholesterol (*low-density* and *very low-density lipoproteins*) and good cholesterol (*high-density lipoproteins*). The bad cholesterol is bad because, after delivering its fat payload, it easily becomes stuck along the internal arterial walls, starting the process of *atherosclerosis*. The good cholesterol has the ability to unstick the cholesterol deposits and bring them back to the liver before these deposits get too hard or calcified. Eating too much fat (very easy to do, if you don't pay attention to your food intake) forces the liver to create more bad cholesterol, thereby reducing your chances of enjoying those extra ten years.

Once the cholesterol has done its dirty work and formed deposits on our artery walls, it is very difficult to reverse the process.

EAT RIGHT

The simplest thing you can do to alter this process is to change the schedule of your eating. According to a study done at the University of Toronto in Canada, cholesterol can be kept in check by eating smaller meals more frequently rather than the same amount of food in less frequent but larger meals. Large meals appear to cause the release of large amounts of insulin, which in turn stimulates the production of an enzyme that increases cholesterol production by the liver. In this study, subjects fed smaller, more frequent meals saw their insulin levels drop by 28 percent, their total cholesterol by 8.5 percent, and their bad cholesterol by 13.5 percent. This illustrates that increasing meal frequency while maintaining constant caloric intake may have a role in the prevention of heart disease.

THE FIBER CONNECTION

The one dietary consideration we hear so much about is the importance of fiber. You've probably also heard about the distinction between soluble and insoluble fiber. Basically, soluble fiber (oatmeal, oat bran, citrus fruits, most beans) dissolves in water and can help by flushing cholesterol out of the small intestine before it can wreak havoc in our cardiovascular system. Some scientists believe that the soluble fiber binds with bile, which aids in digestion, and which contains much cholesterol, so that the cholesterol is quickly eliminated by the body. For those men with high serum cholesterol levels, as little as a cup and a half of beans in our daily diet can lower cholesterol by 60 points, according to one study. In a follow-up study, a 76-point drop occurred in only six months.

The second type of fiber, the insoluble (wheat bran), does not dissolve in water. Its important function is in promoting regularity, thus helping to reduce the risk of colon cancer.

Why Bugs Bunny Has Low Cholesterol

So for reducing cholesterol in your blood, soluble fiber is the key. Most vegetables will provide soluble fiber to remove cholesterol by binding it with bile acids. Medical researchers have found that carrot fiber does this through a substance called calcium pectate, a type of pectin. According to the doctors, it may be possible to lower serum cholesterol "ten to twenty percent just by eating two carrots a day. . . ." Eh, what's up, Doc? Certainly not your cholesterol level.

AVOID SATURATED FATS

Another distinction must be made regarding the different types of dietary fats. There are very specific differences among them, so allow me to clarify.

Bad Fats and Good Fats

The *saturated* fats, found in animal products, are the *bad* fats. These raise blood cholesterol levels and promote heart disease. The *unsaturated* fats, mostly from vegetable sources, are the *okay* fats. But a particular *kind of unsaturated fat*, primarily from deep-water fish, (known as *omega-3s*) are the *good* fats.

Omega-3s—the Best of All

Omega-3s appear to inhibit clotting, and to open the tight pathways of the arteries. Simply put, less blood stickiness and wider arteries mean less opportunity for heart attacks.

A study using omega-3s for patients undergoing angioplasty (a procedure for widening occluded arteries) found that those patients who had 3.2 grams of omega-3s per day in the form of fish-oil capsules had half as many recurring problems as those not having the omega-3s.

In another study, a diet rich in salmon (broiled, baked, in salad and lasagna) offered to nine men for forty days resulted in a 10 percent rise of a type of good cholesterol in their bodies. The omega-3 fatty acids in the fish may help block the production of bad cholesterol in the liver.

In a British study of over 2,000 male heart attack victims, eating two or three portions per week of such fish as salmon, trout, kipper, herring, and sardines revealed that, although they weren't protected against repeat heart attacks, they were 29 percent less likely to die within two years, as compared to a similar group not having the advantage of omega-3s.

Whatever our dietary means of reducing cholesterol, doing so can lengthen our lifespan. By how much exactly, is impossible to say. For high-risk individuals—those who smoke, are overweight, or already have heart problems—this increase in lifespan may be up to one full year. But whether it's one year, two years, or more, controlling cholesterol levels in our bodies is a worthwhile endeavor. As we've seen, this must be done by reducing fat, in addition to the use of cholesterol-lowering drugs.

Reversing Heart Disease

Heart disease begins in childhood. Fact. By adulthood, cholesterol buildup may be closing off as much as 65 percent of the arterial passages. Fact. The rate of buildup can accelerate to fatal heart attacks. Fact. What a dismal outlook! Fortunately, for those of us who choose to live longer, some relatively recent and provocative research offers the promise of reversing the process to some extent. Three separate research programs have explored the possibility of scaling back the cardiovascular effects of an unhealthy lifestyle. Two of these studies used a combination of drugs and low-fat diet. A third study used a holistic approach that included exercise, yoga, meditation, and group support.

Twenty-two Percent-Fat Diet

The first study USC performed looked at 188 nonsmoking men who had undergone bypass surgery. Ninety-four were placed on a 22-percent-fat diet along with colestipol and large doses of niacin. The other half had the benefits of the diet, but not the drugs. The drug-taking group showed a "spectacular reduction" in their total cholesterol, and what was more amazing, 16 percent showed actual decreases in their arterial plaque. Arteries have a remarkable healing ability.

Thirty Percent-Fat Diet

Three groups of men with high cholesterol levels were studied by Dr. Greg Brown at the University of Washington. In a similar procedure, one group was given niacin and colestipol; a second group, colestipol and lovastatin; the third, two placebos (inert sugar pills). All groups were given a diet limited to 30 percent fat. After $2^1/_2$ years, both drug groups experienced large drops in serum cholesterol and 35 percent of these two groups showed a decrease in arterial plaque.

Ten Percent-Fat Diet

The most provocative study was that of Dr. Dean Ornish of UC at San Francisco. His experimental group of men was restricted to a vegetarian diet of less than 10 percent fat and all oils were banned. In addition to the yoga, meditation, and group support sessions, as well as exercise and smoking prohibition, the group was taught stress-management techniques. After a year, 18 of the 22 experimental subjects (82 percent) had a regression of heart blockage, while the control group of 19 men showed deterioration in two-thirds of the group.

A Total Plan for a Healthier Heart

What many find exciting in this research is the role that stress and tension may play in heart disease, and, conversely, how relaxation and group togetherness can affect the blood chemistry to result in a healthier cardiovascular system.

After all is said and research completed, there is no substitute for a multimodal approach. Each element of treatment or prevention contributes its part. For a longer, more youthful life, we need all the help we can muster. Taking control of your health is not a halfway proposition.

1. Eating less red meat, whole milk products, and more fruits and vegetables is essential. Less fats and more fiber is our goal.

2. Although drugs may be necessary in extreme cases only, a daily dosage of 500 mg. of niacin (*not* the timed-release form) along with the rest of our vitamins is a good bet for most of us.

3. Following through on our daily exercise regimen will lower our total cholesterol level and raise the good cholesterol component.

4. Avoiding stress and making our lives more pleasant and enjoyable through group support and healthy, loving relationships helps keep our hearts happy in more ways than we can possibly imagine.

Did you know that if you ate only vegetables and fruit—nothing else—you would have ample protein to keep you healthy and strong?

If, on a particular day, you were to eat two servings of carrots, a few servings of various beans and some summer squash and other assorted veggies of your choice—that is, one day of vegetables only, no fish or fowl—you would have about 30 grams of pure protein in that day's diet.

I don't necessarily recommend that, but I do want to start off making a very strong point: Although some fish, fowl, even occasional red meat in your meals is alright, they're not essential to proper nutrition, especially since you're already getting many of your vitamins and minerals in the supplements just described in Chapter 6.

The most important thing for you to consider is that, to live ten years longer in good health and appearance, you need to transform your attitude toward fatty foods.

Although we are typically attracted to foods containing fat—from gravies to french fries to succulent pastries—we must realize that fat is a dangerous killer. Consider the Surgeon General's Report as well as the report of the Committee on Diet and Health of the National Research Council. There is agreement: Too much fat in the diet is the greatest nutritional hazard in America.

That's not to say you should *never* eat anything with fat. But it *is* to say that these foods should be highly exceptional in your overall eating habits.

Fat Craving Is Natural

There is a theory that the desire for fat is an evolved characteristic. Historically, famines and epidemics of disease affected our ancestors on a regular basis—almost every few years—and those that survived were fat eaters who acquired enough extra weight to survive such regular scourges. Consequently, the desire for fatty foods evolved in the survivors, who eventually gave birth to us. To the extent that this theory is valid, we can forgive ourselves for our craving for fatty foods.

You Mustn't Give in. You mustn't give in to your cravings regularly if you choose to live ten years longer. If you need living proof of this, consider an ongoing, very large-scale "experiment" comparing the lifespans of those who eat a typical amount of fat in their daily food consumption with those who typically avoid fat in their meals.

Seventh-Day Adventists

Such an "experimental" group is the Seventh-Day Adventists, acknowledged in much scientific research to be the single healthiest group of individuals in America. Among the health principles of these individuals is the vegetarian eating style. Although there are varying degrees of adherence to this, as a group, they can be characterized as vegetarians.

RESULTS: VEGETARIANS LIVE LONGER. Scientists have found that, among this group, men live almost nine years longer than their American counterparts, and women live seven and one-half years longer. Both men and women in this group have lower incidences of most forms of cancer. The death rate due to heart disease is roughly half that of the "normal" American population. For those Seventh-Day Adventists who are total vegetarians (no meat, milk, or eggs), the death rate due to heart disease is only 12 percent of the general population!

CHOOSE MORE NATURAL AND LESS PROCESSED FOODS

So, to live ten years longer, a simple shift in values is in order: Decrease the amount of fats in your meals significantly, and increase the proportion of fruits and vegetables radically. The principle is really quite simple; the trick is in being creative in how you present the fruits and vegetables. And keep it simple in terms of avoiding processed foods.

A crisp, delicious apple is only 70 calories. Take that same apple, give it to a food processing company to turn it into all-American apple pie, and that very same apple is now 350 calories.

Processing Foods Increases Calories

A steamy, hearty baked potato is 100 calories. Give that same potato to a fast-food chain to turn into French fries (300 calories) or potato chips (800 calories) and you're on your way to a shorter life. So keeping it simple means doing as little as possible to the original state of the food, except to wash, cut, and occasionally steam or cook.

Be Creative!

Fruits can be mixed together in interesting combinations using crushed nuts as condiments. How about diced pears in a half-cantaloupe sprinkled with raisins and crushed walnuts? And for dessert, some pouty kumquats nestling among a bowl of strawberries and blueberries in a shallow bed of grapefruit juice. The possibilities are endless.

Similarly for vegetables: A wide variety of herbs, seasonings, extracts, and chopped nuts can adorn any dish of steamed vegetables prepared in various combinations.

Feel Full and Stay Thin

The closer you stick to a vegetarian menu (including brown rice and whole grain breads, of course) the more you can look forward to leaving the table with a full stomach, and *still* end up being thin. It's hard to get fat on a vegetarian lifestyle.

Down with Sugar

Aside from drastically reducing the amount of meat in your meals, the next step is to similarly reduce foods high in refined sugar such as cake, pastry, and other foods, such as ice cream, soft drinks, and candy.

Watch out, as well, for hidden fats such as butter on your steamed veggies, and mayonnaise and salad dressings on your salads. These condiments alone can double your fat intake if you're not careful.

Fat-free, Yet Still Delicious

There are many fat-free and sugar-free ways of making food sweet and delicious. Fruit juices can be used as a sweetener instead of refined sugar, with nuts and herbs as condiments. Instead of regular cheese (high in fat), you can buy soy cheese made from organic soy milk that simulates the taste and texture of real cheese. This can be found at most health-food stores.

Soy cheese can top a steamed potato along with sweet basil and dill. For a garden salad, try adding chives, rosemary, lemon, or thyme. For a fruit salad, try lemon balm or coriander. The potential for creativity is endless. Getting thin and living longer through these eating habits can be a lot of fun, especially if you enjoy a creative challenge.

Curing Heart Disease Without Surgery

In his preliminary study, Dr. Ornish found ten volunteers (from a pool of over 10,000 patients) who had documented coronary heart disease and chest pain, but who were not going to have bypass surgery. Once in Dr.Ornish's program, these patients' cholesterol and blood pressure readings began to drop significantly. After only one month, an exercise thallium scan test, measuring blood flow to the heart, showed significant improvements in coronary blood flow.

In his second study, Dr. Ornish and his colleagues studied 48 patients. Half of this group adhered closely to Dr. Ornish's program; the other half followed the advice of their own physicians. While those who followed their own doctors' advice "stayed the same or became slightly worse," those in Dr. Ornish's program enjoyed a 91 percent reduction in chest pain, a 21 percent reduction in cholesterol levels, and a 55 percent improvement in exercise capability. According to Dr. Ornish, "Using a different nuclear medicine test called a gated pool scan, we measured overall improvements both in the ability of the heart to pump blood and in how uniformly it was contracting, two indirect indications that the heart disease was improving after only twenty-four days."

What did Dr. Ornish do to produce such miraculous results? Nothing new! Just a combination of approaches that were put together in a sincerely directed project that involved not only a low-fat diet and exercise, but also a stress-reduction program that provided a great deal of caring and emotional support, as well as yoga, meditation, and visualization.

Become a Creative Vegetarian

Many diets suggest limiting calories by a certain amount. This means counting every time you eat. That won't work because it's just not natural to do so. A much more viable approach is to work toward becoming a vegetarian. Don't worry about counting calories—we've already learned that worrying is bad for you. Instead, as time goes by, learn to enjoy creative ways of eating vegetables, fruit, whole-grain breads, and pastas. Begin to appreciate how toxic highly processed foods are, with their high sugar, salt, and fat contents. You'll lose weight easily. You'll feel better, have more energy, and sleep better.

What's more, you can look forward to living ten years longer if you follow such principles—ten years of looking better, feeling better, and enjoying it all more. It's all available just by getting to the heart of the matter.

THE FRENCH PARADOX

In the fall of 1991, a segment on the CBS news program "60 Minutes" convinced many North American viewers of the benefits of red wine and foie gras in combating heart disease.

It appeared that the French were eating as much fat as Americans and yet experiencing only half as many heart attacks. American TV viewers, alert to new findings on improving their health, immediately went out and, of course, stocked up on red wine and foie gras. According to Information Resources, Inc., of San Francisco, in the eight weeks ending January 12, 1992, sales of red wine in American supermarkets rose to 1,374,000 cases—354,000 more than the 1,020,000 sold in the same period of the preceding 12 months.

Along with everyone else, I was impressed, then somewhat confused by these findings. How could eating larger quantities of a fat-laden food reduce heart disease when all research indicates the opposite?

Upon closer examination, it appears that there really is no inconsistency. Here's why: It takes many years for atherosclerosis to take place—many years of too much fat in the foods eaten daily. So if we were to look at what Frenchmen and women ate ten, twenty, thirty, and forty years ago, what would that reveal? Actually, since the age of susceptibility to heart attacks is typically 50 and above, we should really look at what our Gallic friends were eating in the 1940s and 1950s.

In the years following World War II, France (along with other countries) was in rough shape, to put it bluntly. Food was scarce enough, but especially high-fat foods such as beef and butter. Vegetables, fruit, bread, and small amounts of cheese were the mainstay of the day. It's quite possible, according to Dr. Henry Blackburn, Mayo professor of public health at the University of Minnesota, "that the period of real deprivation in France, in the '40s, would have had something of a protective effect. . . the lag time between the change in fat intake and the appearance of heart disease has been seen in other cultures, including Japan."

"It's quite possible," said the late Dr. Jean Mayer, a nutritionist and past president of Tufts University, "that 20 to 30 years from now the French may have as much heart disease as we do."

Let's look at some figures. According to the United Nations Food and Agriculture Organization, in 1960 the French were getting only 28 percent of their calories from fat. In the United States, on the other hand, this figure was 39 percent in 1940, twenty years earlier. It took France almost three decades to catch up to that figure. By 1988, they were also up to 39 percent; by that time, the U.S. figure was 42 percent. So most likely what we are seeing today in terms of French citizens having fewer heart attacks than Americans is the lower fat figure of decades ago.

According to Dr. Marion Nestle, a nutritionist at New York University, "The French diet is newly high in fat, and heart disease rates just haven't had time to catch up. . . . We have had 40 to 50 years of a food supply at least this high in fat, compared to three to five years for France. No wonder their heart disease rates are lower."

So if you've already stocked up on foie gras and red wine, go ahead and enjoy it—only *very* moderately. What we see in this chapter is that to nurture a healthy heart, and even cure one that is already sick with occluded arteries, we need the three legs of a healthy tripod:

1. Moderate exercise.
2. Self-esteem buoyed by an emotionally supportive network.
3. A 10 percent-fat food intake.

REDUCE SALT AND INCREASE POTASSIUM

As if cholesterol problems weren't enough, another area of concern, if we are to earn ten years more in our lives, is that of high blood pressure. This is medically defined as beginning at 140/90 mm. Hg (the number of millimeters a column of mercury rises as a result of the pressure). The first number is referred to as the systolic pressure, during the moment of heart contraction. The second number, the diastolic pressure, occurs during the heart's resting phase between beats.

Just Lowering Your Blood Pressure Will Get You Ten More Years

The problem with high blood pressure is that it aggravates the cholesterol problems, creates problems in general for the cardiovascular system by increasing the resistance against which the heart must pump, and most hazardous of all, it predisposes the individual to a greater risk of stroke (a break in a blood vessel in the brain due to too much pressure against a weakened vessel wall). Middle-aged men with hypertension are three times more likely to suffer a heart attack and seven times more likely to suffer from a stroke. Their lives may be shortened by an average of ten to twenty years. So if you suffer from high blood pressure, just bringing it back to normal may give you the ten years I've been promising you. Let's get to work!

Drugs for lowering blood pressure are ineffective unless taken for an entire lifetime. Although antihypertensive drugs will lower blood pressure, that effect is available only while the drugs are being taken. In other words, they must be taken for life. A large-scale study of 612 people in Helsinki revealed that although the drugs resulted in a 35 percent reduction in blood pressure, *the participants developed twice as much heart disease* after five years when compared with the control group of patients who took fewer antihypertensive and cholesterol-lowering drugs! Drugs are not the answer to lifelong cardiovascular problems.

Down with Salt

For about one-fourth to one-third of those suffering from hypertension, sodium (as in sodium chloride—common table salt) seems to play an important role. Unless you definitely know you're not in that category, you need to start reducing your salt intake. A low-salt, low-calorie diet alone may be sufficient to normalize your blood pressure.

Reducing your salt intake may appear easier than it really is. The first step, the easy one, is never to use a salt shaker. The harder one is avoiding the hidden salt used in cooking and processing foods. In our preindustrial days, we probably consumed no more than 0.5 g. of salt (less than one-eighth teaspoon) per day. The average American now consumes between 7 and 15 g. of salt per day, at least fifteen times as much. No wonder our collective blood pressure is soaring.

Back to Nature

As we age, it is commonly expected that our blood pressure increases. But that is likely because of the salt that has come along with our industrialized status. Dr. Hugh Trowell, in a letter to the *British Medical Journal*, wrote that among primitive hunter gatherers who add no salt to their food, "blood pressures do not rise with age, and essential hypertension is virtually unknown."

Watch Out for Hidden Salt

Processed foods are notorious for the amount of hidden salt they contain, including almost all TV dinners, canned soups, luncheon meats, and condiments such as ketchup and mustard. So it pays to be vigilant. The more natural, unprocessed foods in your diet, the better off you are all around.

Up with Potassium

The other element under discussion, potassium, has just the opposite effect. An increase of this in our diet seems to improve our blood pressure readings.

Just as some people's cardiovascular systems are sensitive to salt, others are similarly sensitive to potassium. In its *absence*, their blood pressure goes up. Dr. George Meneely spent three decades studying the sodium/potassium levels in rats and concluded that increased potassium levels could greatly extend their lifespan. "In nature, there is a relatively small amount of sodium in any diet and there is much more potassium than sodium in *all* natural diets," explains Dr. Meneely.

Vegetables Have Good Minerals

Vegetarians, who tend to have lower blood pressure and cholesterol levels, owe this benefit to the higher levels of minerals—magnesium, calcium, and potassium—in their diet.

A research design to show the effects of low potassium intake was done by Dr. Gopal Krishna at the Temple University School of Medicine. Ten men with normal blood pressure were fed two different diets—one with normal amounts of potassium, the other low in potassium. Sodium remained the same normal amount for both. After only nine days, the diastolic pressure of the low potassium group went from 91 to 95. Sodium and fluid retention also rose. Dr. Krishna speculates that the resulting high sodium level may induce hypertension.

Balance Minerals to Extend Life Expectancy Thirty Percent

The key to avoiding or correcting high blood pressure seems to lie in maintaining the right balance in our daily nutrition. Maintaining a healthy cardiovascular system for life is simple and straightforward. As Dr. James Scala puts it, ". . . with a little effort we can extend life expectancy 30 percent simply by applying the knowledge we already have."

The K Factor

Dr. Scala knows whereof he speaks. In his book, *High Blood Pressure Relief Diet*, he explains how natural, unprocessed foods come high in potassium (K), while processed foods come high in sodium (Na). The K factor of a food is simply the K/Na ratio. For good vascular health, we need much more K than Na in our systems. According to Dr. Scala, "Medical scientists are recognizing more and more that a dietary K factor of 3 or more is essential to optimum health. The problem of too much dietary sodium cannot be overstated."

How It Works. To illustrate how the K factor works, let's apply it to some common foods. A typical serving of corn flakes provides a K factor of 0.07. Not very healthy. A slice of roast beef has a K factor of 12. Quite healthy, if you didn't have to worry about the high level of fat and cholesterol. A hot dog has a K factor of 0.15. Terrible for your blood pressure as well as your cholesterol. Now, for an interesting comparison, let's compare a simple apple in its natural form with a slice of frozen apple pie.

Apple—GOOD! Apple Pie—BAD!

A simple apple contains 159 mg. of K to only 1 mg. of Na, for a K factor of 159. Terrific! That'll go a long way to help us get an average above 3. The apple pie, on the other hand, contains 73 mg. of K to 298 mg. of Na for a K factor of 0.24. What a difference! This illustrates dramatically what happens when we take a simple, healthy food and process it to the point of being close to toxic. According to Dr. Scala, ". . . when the dietary potassium to sodium ratio—the K factor—falls below 3 to about 1 or even 1.5, high blood pressure increases dramatically." Writes Dr. Scala:

> Natural foods . . . contain much more potassium than sodium. Indeed, the ratio in animal foods of 3 is low compared to vegetables, where the ratio is often 10 or more. . . . In fact, estimates by some anthropologists place the potassium to sodium ratio in the diet of our remote ancestors of 10,000 years ago at about 16!. . .So, if we lived in harmony with nature, our K factor would be 3 or more.

A simple baked potato, with no added condiments, has a powerful K factor of 130. Other great K factor foods are fresh fruits and vegetables, beans, rice, and grains.

Fast Foods—VERY BAD!

On the other hand, watch out for the hidden sodium in convenience and fast foods. A McDonald's Big Mac has 950 mg. of sodium. A

Burger King Whopper with cheese has a whopping 1,164 mg. of sodium. Even your drinking water may harbor hidden sodium. A 1981 study revealed that 42 percent of the nation's water supply exceeded the EPA's recommendation of 20 mg./liter.

Boiling vegetables, too, leaches away a good portion of their potassium. As an alternative, try baking, steaming, or microwaving.

TAKE ANTIOXIDANTS AND NIACIN

Other than soluble fiber and omega-3 fatty acids, two more substances worthy of consideration are beta-carotene, an antioxidant found in fruits and vegetables, particularly those of orange or reddish coloring such as carrots and sweet potatoes, and such vitamins as E and niacin (B_3).

Beta-carotene

Beta-carotene, discussed in Chapter 6, converts to vitamin A in the body. Cholesterol builds up not only on arterial walls, but also *inside* the cells of the artery wall. Only oxidized cholesterol is built up in the arteries. By preventing oxidation of the bad cholesterol through dietary antioxidants such as beta-carotene and vitamin E, the bad cholesterol is prevented from being taken up.

Niacin: the "Safe" Drug

Another vitamin that has a strong track record of effectiveness in lowering cholesterol hazards is niacin or vitamin B_3. Niacin, in daily doses of at least 500 mg., has the effect of lowering both total cholesterol and the bad cholesterol component, but also of raising the level of the good cholesterol component. To its credit, niacin has the best track record for safety of all cholesterol-lowering drugs and is the least expensive by far. The wholesale cost for a year's supply of niacin is about $50. Other cholesterol-lowering agents would cost anywhere from $375 (gemfibrozil or probucol) to $910 (lovastatin).

Niacin: The "Poor" Drug

Despite this, niacin has a bad reputation for two reasons. First, since drug companies don't make much of a profit off niacin (compared to gemfibrozil, lovastatin, and so on), niacin falls through the cracks of medical advertising. Most physicians are much more likely to prescribe the more expensive (and less safe) medications.

Avoid the Timed-Release Form

Second, the few cases of serious side effects have been heavily publicized. Of the thousands upon thousands of people taking niacin, only about a couple of dozen individuals have had problems with temporary cases of liver dysfunction, and these only on timed-release forms. In one report, three people taking 2,000 to 4,000 mg. of timed-release niacin daily had only mild hepatitis, and all returned to normal when they returned to regular niacin. Why? "We speculate that regular niacin is only in the blood for a short time," according to Dr. Yaakov Henkin of the University of Alabama, "so it allows liver enzymes to recuperate, while timed-release niacin does not." In any case, I recommend that a doctor's supervision is appropriate for an ongoing regimen of daily dosages of over 500 mg. It's worth the effort. The proper dosage of B_3 can lower cholesterol by 11 percent in men under 50, and by 22 percent in older men.

EXERCISE, STOP SMOKING, AND REDUCE STRESS

Reducing cholesterol through medication and eating less fat will reduce the risk of heart disease, but there is more to be done beyond that. An arduous review of the medical literature reveals that cholesterol-lowering drugs, along with stress-reduction techniques, can lower cholesterol levels already built up in the arterial walls and improve life expectancy. Fat and cholesterol in food need to be reduced if we are to live longer, of course, but here are the additional steps you need to take:

1. Continue the dietary guidelines for thinness (Chapter 6).

2. Avoid saturated fats from animal products such as lard, butter, and meat, as well as products processed with coconut or palm oil (for example, most crackers and many fast foods).

3. Continue to exercise on a routine basis (Chapter 7).

4. Take your vitamins (Chapter 6).

5. Give up caffeine.

6. Stop smoking (Chapter 10).

7. Reduce the stress in your life.

One interesting sidelight to Dr. Ornish's research was the absence of any correlation between blood cholesterol levels and the degree of change in cholesterol deposits in the arteries, an indication that we may be overestimating the importance of cholesterol readings. Says Dr. Ornish: "I am becoming increasingly convinced that other factors, including emotional stress, perceived isolation, lack of social support, hostility, cynicism, and low self-esteem also play important roles."

In the following section, we'll take a look at the growing awareness of how social and emotional factors play a significant role in preventing heart disease.

BUILD A NETWORK OF EMOTIONAL SUPPORT

An effective component of Dr. Ornish's program lies in stress management. According to the good doctor:

> Anything that promotes a sense of isolation leads to chronic stress and often to illnesses like heart disease. Conversely, anything that leads to real intimacy and feelings of connection can be healing in the real sense of the word: to bring together, to make whole. The ability to be intimate has long been seen as a key to emotional health; I believe it is essential to the health of our hearts as well.

Dr. Ornish describes two forms of intimacy—*horizontal* and *vertical*:

Horizontal intimacy can be increased through participation in support groups, development of communication skills, learning forgiveness, developing feelings of trust, practicing altruism, and so on. Prayer and meditation are two ways of realizing *vertical intimacy*—developing the connections between us and the higher parts of ourselves.

After reviewing over a dozen research studies revealing how supportive and caring relationships help protect us from heart disease, Dr. Ornish concludes: "The self-involvement, hostility, and cynicism that predispose us to heart disease are really effects of a more fundamental cause: the perception of isolation."

This was confirmed in three separate, large-scale studies involving almost 7,000 individuals in Alameda County, California; over 2,000 individuals in Evans County, Georgia; and over 13,000 individuals in eastern Finland. Independent of other cardiac risk factors such as cholesterol and blood pressure readings, those who were socially isolated were two to three times as likely to die than those who had strong emotional ties with others. A seven-year study of Hawaiian residents of Japanese ancestry revealed that social networks provided protection against heart attacks, chest pain, and coronary heart disease.

A number of smaller-scale studies had similar findings. A study of 331 elderly people in Durham County, North Carolina showed that those who did not have much social support were four times as likely to die than those who did. A Swedish study of 150 middle-aged men showed that social isolation was one of the best predictors of mortality. And finally, a study of 256 healthy senior citizens in Wisconsin showed that those with good social support systems tended to have lower blood cholesterol readings and better immune functioning.

These studies taken together obviously make a powerful statement. Beyond a 10 percent-fat diet and the proper amount of physical exercise, emotional support appears to be the third leg in this tripod of elements providing the basis of reversing heart disease, and lengthening your life a good ten years.

As I was researching the work of Dr. Ornish in preparation for this book, I viewed a videotape of his research in which the participants were followed through their daily lives to illustrate the integration of the program's principles. One of the participants was a highly competitive athlete who nonetheless was suffering from blocked coronary arteries. This individual, Sam, was fulfilling every component of Dr. Ornish's program, save one. He kept his fats under 10 percent, he exercised furiously, but he could not get himself to open up emotionally. He'd sit in group meetings with his arms folded across his chest. If ever he was emotionally touched by others' sharing, all he'd utter was: "Well, I used to have that problem, but not any more."

Although Sam kept to his dietary commitment and was running and cycling over a hundred miles a week, he would not open his heart to the support network. Sam died.

He was on a rowing machine connected to a video which displayed competing rowboats. Sam was determined to be victorious. He rowed and rowed and rowed for more than an hour, working feverishly to excel against a machine. Sam won, the machine lost. Then Sam died.

As I watched the videotape, Sam's death hit me hard. I'm not one to come easily to tears, but tears did come. What a waste! All this excellent effort, wonderful care, sophisticated medical technology, but the wall around Sam's heart was inviolable. Despite all the care surrounding him, Sam was ultimately a lonely, alienated individual. His heart was starved of caring, and died, leaving those loving friends around him the wiser for it.

I was amazed at the irony of how one individual's death could affect me so much more profoundly than the thousands who were studied by scientists to come up with the very same finding—loneliness kills!

AGE-PROOFING
YOUR SKIN AND HAIR

CHAPTER

9

The sun shone brightly on graduation day as students and faculty convened for the ceremony at Georgia State University. Three hundred and sixty summer graduates and their family members were eager to hear the words of wisdom from media mogul Ted Turner, president of Turner Broadcasting System and winner of sailing's highest honor, the America's Cup.

"The one piece of advice I can give you," stated the candid and outspoken self-made man, "is to put on sunscreen and wear a hat." After a stunned silence, Turner confided to his audience, "I'm going straight from here to a skin cancer operation."

Although a very hard worker, Turner also spent a good deal of time outdoors, honing his sailing skills, trout fishing for relaxation, and watching his successful Atlanta Braves from private seats near the dugout. All that sun without sunscreen at the Southern latitude of Atlanta finally took its toll.

Turner is undoubtedly more aware than ever before, more aware of the possibilities of keeping his skin not only cancer-free, but younger looking by ten years as well. In this chapter, you too can become much more aware of such possibilities.

As we reach for ten more youthful years, it would be helpful to have an overview of the changes in our appearance that normally take place as we age. The healthier we live, the more slowly we age, but the process goes on nonetheless. Not only do we want to live ten years longer, but we want to stay as young-looking as possible throughout our life. In this chapter, we'll chart the changes that take place in our skin and our hair and teeth, along with suggestions on how to deal with them.

Our caveman ancestors were lucky to survive into their 20s. When Columbus sailed the ocean blue, Europeans were happy to reach the then ripe old age of 40. Although Göethe lived into his 80s and Beethoven lived to the age of 56, most of their contemporaries were happy to reach the age of 50. In the next 60 years, our life expectancy could jump another ten years. If we simply reduce deaths from cancer and heart disease, says medical demographer Jay Olshansky of the Argonne National Labs in Chicago, life expectancy could jump from 75 to 85 by the year 2050. That means 30 million people 85 and older by 2050. Let's make sure we can stay youthful-looking throughout such longer lifespans.

"We would not be able to extend the quantity of life without extending the quality as well," says George Roth of the National Institute on Aging. One way of doing this is by the judicious use of such drugs as Deprenyl, human growth hormone and nerve growth factor, but these are still in the research stage and it usually turns out that each drug has its own list of side effects. A much safer approach is to deal with each aspect of aging in a specific way which aims at that particular change as it occurs. So let's look at skin in its own light. But first an overview, from head to toe.

There are ways to care for the skin as the sensitive organ it is. Yet this chapter offers no miracles, no magic bullets. Rather, it explores what can age the skin by neglect: overexposure to the sun, lack of proper hygiene, poor diet, and substance abuse. It also explores what men can and cannot do in order to ageproof their skin.

YOUR SKIN AS YOU AGE

The skin is an organ covering your entire body and made up of two basic layers, the underlying *dermis* and the outer *epidermis*, comprised from inside out of the basal or germinative layer, the *stratum spinosum*, the *stratum granulosum*, and the horny outer covering that is visible. The *stratum corneum* itself is made up of 15 to 20 layers of cells.

Transit Time

New skin cells are formed at the basal layer, starting off round and plump. They then travel through the next three levels, getting older and flatter as they go, until they reach the outer, visible layer where they're prepared to be shed or scraped off. Dermatologists refer to the time it takes for this trip through the four layers as *transit time*, and the process of shedding is called *desquamation*. If the cells are scraped off, as in scrubbing, this is often referred to as *exfoliation*.

As you can now see, the skin is a very active organ, hardly resting for a moment, though it looks very inactive to the uninformed observer.

Why You Look Older as You Age

As you get older, the transit time slows down. The transit time of an 80-year-old is four to six weeks, as compared to that of a 20-year-old, whose transit time is merely two to three weeks. The longer it takes the skin cells to get to the outer layer, the older and flatter the cells are when they get there. So it's no wonder that older men look older.

Even as you enter your 30s, cell turnover begins to slow down, making your skin look somewhat duller. Your years of exposure to the sun begin to give you those fine furrows and laugh lines. Your skin begins to behave like a little garden, sprouting small red "domes" known as cherry angiomas, and benign brown or grayish raised tumors, known as seborrheic keratoses.

How Midlife Affects Your Skin

As you enter your 40s, your skin begins to thin out ever so slightly, making it more susceptible to the harmful effects of the sun. Gravity starts to take dominion over your face as the skin loses some of its elasticity, causing noticeable sagging at the eyes and jowls. You may begin to show more "character," not to mention occasional discoloration of the skin. As you go quietly into mid-life, your skin becomes drier, especially in the cold, windy climates with less moisture in the air. To battle, gentlemen!

SIX STEPS TO YOUNGER SKIN

So how to keep your skin from aging? Here are six sure-fire ways to keep skin ten years younger. The remainder of the chapter will fill in the details of these six steps so you can do each one properly.

1. Avoid overexposure to the sun
   - ❏ wear sunscreen
   - ❏ apply generously and reapply as often as needed
   - ❏ wear a broad-rimmed hat in the sun
   - ❏ wear protective clothing
   - ❏ exercise outdoors primarily in mornings or evenings

2. Avoid tobacco and excess alcohol

3. Accelerate your skin's transit time
   - ❏ choose a gentle exfoliating technique
     - scrubs
     - cleansing grains

4. Moisturize your skin
   - ❏ drink your fill of water
   - ❏ apply moisturizing ointments

5. Feed your skin properly
   - ❏ vitamins A, B, C, and E are critical for youthful appearance

6. Procedures your doctor can prescribe or perform
   - ❏ chemical peel
   - ❏ dermabrasion
   - ❏ Retin-A

HOW TO PROTECT YOUR SKIN FROM THE SUN

Victor was a minister in his mid-40s who enjoyed gardening as his hobby. He labored lovingly over his exotic flowers on a daily basis under the bright Georgia sun, taking satisfaction in the tan he always had.

One day he noticed a raw spot on the side of his face right in front of his right ear. It would not go away. A doctor's visit confirmed his worst fear—skin cancer. Luckily, it was easily removable. But from then on Victor was much more conscious of the damaging effect of the sun's rays. Victor, like many other men, was completely ignorant about the potential damage that the sun can have on a man's skin.

By far, the most important aspect of keeping your skin ten years younger is avoiding overexposure to the sun. I shudder whenever I see young people "catching some rays" with a hand-held reflector. They're usually in their twenties or early thirties. By the time they're in their late thirties and forties and start to notice wrinkles and "liver spots" for the first time, they're more likely to be sensible about sun exposure. The "Hollywood tan," lasting only a few days, is an expensive price to pay for temporary glamour. And the price isn't paid till years later, when wrinkled skin cannot be reversed to the smoothness of skin undamaged by sun.

Loss of smoothness is only one aspect of sun damage. Radiation-damaged skin shows pigment variation (light and dark patches/mottling), thinning of the epidermis, yellowing, fine beading, and *telangiectasia* (blood vessel/capillary enlargement)—seen as red lines, fan-like, or branching. Sunburn is a precursor to tanning in those who can tan. The darker your natural skin tone, the less easily you will burn. Some people just burn and tan very little, if at all—especially very fair, red-headed, freckled, blue-eyed folks.

"Sunlight is the single most devastating factor in hastening aging skin," according to Dr. Tom Sternberg, UCLA dermatologist. "For sunlight affects all the layers including the top subcutaneous layer in producing sagging and wrinkling. . . . It is *cumulative, permanent,* and *progressive.*" As much as 80 percent of the visible signs of aging are directly due to sun exposure.

Jog or Walk in the Early AM or Late PM

So if you're going to jog or walk as your form of exercise, it would be wise to do it in the morning or late afternoon, or after sunset if possible. One of the few benefits of living in Southern California or Denver or other smog-infested areas lies in the fact that the dirty air acts as a bit of a filter by absorbing sunburn-producing rays. The silver lining of the cloud of smog may help protect you from damaging sunlight, but you're strongly advised to do all you can to protect yourself. "Beware of cloudy days," warns Dr. Harvey Finkelstein, a Canadian dermatologist. "You can still burn, as much radiation still impinges on the skin via the phenomenon of 'scattering'."

How Sunscreens Work

In addition to the obvious clothing and hats that protect the skin of your body and face, there's the option of sunscreens. Basically, these fall into three categories: *absorbers, reflectors,* and a *combination of the two.* Absorbers have *para-aminobenzoic acid* (PABA) or related compounds as an essential ingredient. These must be absorbed into the skin to be effective. This type of sunscreen is typically clear and may include cinnamates, digalloy trioleate, pyrones and salicylates. The PABA absorbs *ultraviolet light*-B (UVB), while the benzophenones cover a wider spectrum of light waves. The anthranilates in sunscreens are moderately effective against both *ultraviolet light*-A (UVA) as well as UVB. State-of-the-art sunscreens contain *Parsol*, generically known as *arobenzone*, which is the best UVA blocker now available—much better in the UVA range than any of the previously developed chemicals.

Reflectors, or physical sunscreens, scatter or reflect ultraviolet rays. These chemicals are made up of red petrolatum or titanium dioxide, zinc oxide, or talc.

Watch Out for UVA Waves

Sun rays are comprised of wavelengths A, B, or C. Ultraviolet light-A waves are responsible only for short-term tanning during the first 24 hours, but penetrate deeply into the dermis and can cause long-term damage. Such UVA waves provide the immediate color change noticed on the first day. Tanning studios which primarily provide UVA (damaging in its own right) may not protect from burns despite the acquisition of a "base" before a summer vacation. These longer, low-energy waves used to be of little concern, but more recently their potential for harm has been a great consideration for manufacturers of sunscreens.

How Sunlight Affects Your Skin

The UVB waves are shorter, higher energy rays that do cause longer-term tanning and sunburn. They do so by stimulating melanocytes to make more melanin in the skin. In addition to affecting the superficial layers of the skin (the stratum granulosum), they deliver ultraviolet to the stratum corneum, the top layers of the skin. These UVB waves are strongest between 10:00 A.M. and 3:00 P.M. The shortest wavelength rays, UVC, are absorbed by the ozone layer in the earth's upper atmosphere. There is a great deal of controversy about whether our concerns about depletion of this ozone layer are realistic or not. Some say our fears are based on inadequate data and merely reflect one isolated segment in an ongoing cyclic pattern; others say ozone depletion is extremely critical and irreversible. In the absence of more certainty, only we as individuals can take responsibility to protect ourselves. Hence, the importance of the sun protection factor.

Things have changed since the sun-worshipping '50s when young men might have used a sun reflector to multiply the tanning effect of the sun. Remember the Coppertone ads encouraging a better tan on the beach in the early '60s? A UVB blocker was the prime ingredient in Coppertone then, giving free reign to the UVA and UVC rays, resulting in the frightening increase in skin cancer among the Baby Boomer Generation (most of us). It takes a number of decades for the accumulated effect of sun damage to show itself. If only we had known then what we know now!

What Is Meant by SPF?

The sun protection factor (SPF) is an index of degrees of protection in sunscreens against exposure to UVB rays, ranging from 2 to 50. Most dermatologists believe an SPF of higher than 15 or 20 doesn't provide any significant increase in protection. A minimum SPF of 15 should be used. But since it doesn't hurt to use a sunscreen with a higher SPF, and since sunscreens can easily lose their potency through perspiration and rubbing against objects or clothing, using higher SPFs is a form of insurance. Better to have more if it doesn't hurt rather than have just enough that's easily removed. Although some sunscreens are prepared to be waterproof and are quite effective when tested after 20 minutes of swimming, no sunscreen is *completely* waterproof.

How Is SPF Determined?

In case you're wondering, the SPF is arrived at by dividing the amount of time you can safely stay out in the sun with a sunscreen, by the amount of time you can safely stay out in the sun without a sunscreen. If you normally get sunburned after 15 minutes of intense sun, a sunscreen with an SPF of 10 will allow you to remain under that same sun for 150 minutes before you get burned. But don't sit in the sun longer because you're wearing a sunscreen. It should *not* be used as a reason to sit and work on your tan without fear of burning. All tans are bad. They reflect radiation injury. No sunscreen is perfect (unless it's opaque). Think of the sunscreen as helping to protect you from solar injury that would otherwise occur if you wore nothing to protect yourself.

Five Danger Points

It's important to remember to apply sunscreens one a half-hour prior to exposure, unless you're using a physical sunscreen such as zinc oxide or titanium dioxide. Don't be stingy when applying it. The SPFs are based on liberal applications. Better to be safe and sloppy than sorry and scarred. Also, if you're swimming or perspiring, don't forget to reapply at regular intervals. Be especially careful if any of the following apply:

1. You're spending a lot of time in or on the water (swimming, water skiing, boating).

2. You're on the beach anywhere near the equator.

3. You're at a high altitude (for example, mountain climbing) where there is less atmosphere to absorb the sun's rays—or near the North Pole (no ozone layer).

4. It's summertime and between 10:00 A.M. and 3:00 P.M.

5. There's enough snow on the ground to reflect the sun.

For Swimmers Only

No matter what your skin shading, color, or race, you still need to protect your skin from the sun. Even black skin needs protection from UVA. If your aerobic activity is outdoor swimming, you're under the sun on a routine basis and it's especially important to protect your skin. So it's important to know the difference between *water-resistant* (good for 40 minutes of swimming) and *waterproof* (good for 80 minutes). But no matter how good a sunscreen is, once it's wiped off (by your arm or a towel), it ceases to perform its function. So if you accidentally wipe some off, be sure to reapply. Looking ten years younger means keeping your skin safe from the most obvious villain: Old Sol in the sky.

What to Wear to Avoid Sun Damage

In addition to sunscreens, there is a whole new line of SPF clothing to help keep your skin below the neck looking ten years younger. A soft, lightweight fabric is made from nylon-based fiber woven to provide an SPF of at least 30 (actually testing as high as 70). For swimming activities, there's a slightly stretchy version. One particular nylon product is coated with an inert, nontoxic chemical and is able to block out 99 percent of UVB and 93 percent of UVA rays. Continued washings do not reduce the sunscreen effect. The FDA has already begun to approve these garments.

Protecting Your Eyes

The eyes can be affected a number of ways as we age. You're probably tired of me going on and on about the harmful effects of the sun, but here we go again. Many elderly men begin to have trouble seeing clearly because of cataracts, a painless clouding of the eye lens. The risk of cataracts is increased by a lifetime of exposure to UVB rays.

If you must be out in the sun a lot, whether driving or exercising, the obvious protection is sunglasses. But the decision as to which glasses to buy is not a simple one. There are many factors to be considered, but the main one is that the glasses protect you from UVB waves.

HOW TO EVALUATE AND OBTAIN THE PROPER SUNGLASSES. In 1986, the American National Standards Institute categorized the effectiveness of sunglasses into three categories: *Cosmetic*—blocking 70 percent of UVB rays and 60 percent of UVA; *general purpose*—blocking 95 percent of UVB and 60 percent of UVA; and *special purpose*—blocking 99 percent of UVB and 98.5 percent of UVA. Problem is that it's difficult to comparison shop because this information is not always available to the consumer. Fortunately for us, a number of sunglasses have been professionally evaluated for their sun-protective effectiveness. Check with your local opticians for guidance in this matter.

One other factor to keep in mind when purchasing your sunglasses—Australian researchers suggest you get wraparound shades to keep the sun's rays from sneaking in through the corners.

One More Reason to Avoid the Sun

The sun, as I've said before, is the single most culpable agent in aging your skin. But there's yet another reason, one we're fairly unfamiliar with. We'll probably learn more about it as time goes by. Apparently, too much sun can weaken the immune system. Studies have shown that UVB rays (most plentiful in the summertime) affect both animals and humans by inhibiting the immune system. Researchers at the M.D. Anderson Cancer Center in Houston report that even chemical sunscreens can't prevent this effect, so all the more reason to watch out for sunburn.

CLEANSING YOUR SKIN FOR LASTING YOUTH

One way of looking ten years younger is to speed up the transit time, so younger looking cells will appear on the surface. Wouldn't it be nice if you could do it?

Well, you can! All it requires is proper hygiene and the strategic use of a washcloth and the proper cleansing agent. Using a scrub or cleansing grains will induce more rapid desquamation and in many individuals will accelerate the transit time, resulting in "newer" cells at the stratum corneum, the outermost, visible layer. You can also, very gently, scrub all over your face, being especially gentle around the corners of your eyes, where it is most advisable to pat rather than scrub.

What kind of cleanser should you scrub with? Well, you can go the natural route and use a handful of cornmeal or oatmeal from your kitchen, or you can go the commercial route and purchase products referred to as cleansing grains, scrub cleansers, sloughing cleansers, or washing grains. These usually consist of abrasive particles—natural ones such as apricot seeds, almonds or oatmeal, or synthetic ingredients such as silica or zirconium oxide—suspended in a cleansing cream. Scrubs for dry skin may include moisturizers or oils. And there are scrubs for oily skin.

The Horny Layer

A gentle scrub will remove the old, dead cells on the top layer of the stratum corneum, otherwise known as the horny layer. Given the bright, fresh look of your scrubbed skin, it just might make your mate feel "horny" toward you.

New Skin

Not only will you look fresh and youthful, the exfoliation encourages and stimulates the formation of new skin cell generation from the basal layer, accelerating the transit time to a more youthful rate.

How Much Does It Cost? Up to You!

This scrubbing method will cost as little or as much as you like. The least expensive involves the use of oatmeal or cornmeal from your kitchen. The most expensive can be found at cosmetic shops. Just so long as it reduces the transit time and keeps your skin youthful.

GETTING RID OF WRINKLES

Randy, a 45-year-old financial advisor, had sported a beard since his 20s. When he finally decided to cut it off, his friends were somewhat surprised by the number of wrinkles now apparent that had been hidden by his beard. Randy had made a decision to give up bachelorhood for marriage—all he needed was an eligible wife. But all his wrinkles were scaring off the "woman of his dreams."

Successful in his profession, Randy was ready to pay the price for a younger look. What were the options available, he asked me.

Welcome the plastic surgeons and dermatologists and their youth-enhancing procedures! If you have the time and money, you can choose from a number of options to bring about some radical changes to enhance your youthful appearance. This is not a philosophical or moral issue (whether or not to tamper with nature), but rather an aesthetic and economic issue.

We spend anywhere from $1,000 to $100,000 for four wheels and a frame to convey us from place to place. We spend anywhere from $50,000 to $2,000,000 (and higher) to keep the rain from falling on our heads. Is it appropriate to consider spending a relatively meager amount to look (and thereby become to all the world around us) as young as your body feels? Although I personally have not afforded myself such a luxury to date, at a philosophical level, I see no reason to avoid contemplating such options.

During your 40s, you may begin to consider chemical peels or dermabrasion after consulting your plastic surgeon or dermatologist. Never do it without a medical doctor trained in this area. Your doctor can also help you with any other skin problems, of course, such as growths. If you want to consider Retin-A, then talk with him or her about that too.

Dermabrasion

The first of these is relatively inexpensive. Dermabrasion can be described as a more intense version of the scrub mentioned earlier in this chapter. Typically, a surgeon uses an instrument like a dental burr to abrade the surface of the skin, accomplished in his office using local anesthesia. This procedure can improve heavily aged skin and is helpful as well in the treatment of acne rosacea.

The dermabrasion procedure goes beneath the horny layer down to the middle layers. As a result, a crust forms on the treated area, coming off after about a week. The area remains red and extremely sensitive for the next two to four weeks. The hope is that this procedure will shorten the transit time of cell generation through to the outer layers, resulting in younger, "plumper" cells at the surface. This is a very delicate procedure, occasionally resulting in scar tissue. So it is advisable to be very careful with this procedure.

Chemical Peel

Chemical peel, also referred to as superficial chemosurgery or skin peeling, consists of applying an acid to the skin, causing the superficial layer to peel away, revealing a smoother, more youthful layer. At one time, carbolic acid or phenol was used, but this substance proved too toxic. Then trichloroacetic acid was used. More currently, such chemicals as the traditional sulfur and salicylic acid lotions as well as the popular benzoyl peroxide and the controversial *tretinoin* (*Retin*-A) are more fashionable.

Retin-A

An early study of Retin-A involved its application on the skin of 30 subjects ranging in age from mid-life to 70. At first, nearly all the subjects suffered from skin inflammation for a period of 2 to 20 weeks. For most, though, once the irritation subsided, Retin-A was found to decrease fine wrinkling and give the skin a healthier, more youthful appearance.

Anyone who uses Retin-A should use a sunscreen when outdoors. Using it without a sunscreen is not only irritating to the skin but may actually accelerate premature aging and increase the risk of skin cancer.

Retin-A actually transforms the skin to a more youthful stage when it does work successfully. A dermatologist at the University of Pennsylvania was one of the first to pioneer its use to renew aging skin. Until then it was used primarily against acne. Retin-A not only accelerates transit time, but also stimulates blood vessel growth in the skin and boosts production of collagen and elastin, both of which decrease with the process of aging. The result? A skin with fewer wrinkles, which can make you look a good ten years younger.

Retin-A has become very popular since its wrinkle-removing effect was discovered over a decade ago. Over the years it's developed a strong reputation for doing a good job. Tretinoin is the active ingredient in both Retin-A and its oilier version, called *Renova*. It has the effect of restoring and revitalizing skin that has been broken down by too much sun exposure. Collagen and elastin fibers in the dermis become more prevalent, and blood flow between the layers of the skin increases. Pinker and smoother skin with fewer wrinkles and lighter age spots can occur with this treatment.

One new, exciting finding about tretinoin is that it actually fights against cancer, reversing the process toward health. In 1993, researchers at the University of Pennsylvania applied Retin-A to one side of the backs of patients with irregular moles that often turn cancerous. After 6 months, the treated side showed smaller moles which were no longer precancerous while the moles on the other side remained unchanged.

KEEPING YOUR SKIN SMOOTH AND CLEAR

In addition to Retin-A, facial scrubs, dermabrasion, and chemical peels, there are also the options of alpha-hydroxy acids, bleaches, and collagen, fibrin or fat injections.

Alpha-hydroxy acids (AHA) come in the form of creams and lotions applied to the skin, generally twice a day. They're primarily moisturizers but may also smooth out fine wrinkles and roughness. Sold by prescription (Lac-Hydrin) or over the counter in weaker form (Alpha Hydrox, Lac-Hydrin Five, Anew), AHA falls somewhere between Retin-A and ordinary moisturizers in effectiveness. This chemical works by speeding up the rate of exfoliation, which slows down with age. It makes the skin look smoother and younger.

The smallest of the AHA molecules penetrate easily and deeply into the skin. Alpha-hydroxy acids may actually produce more collagen, a structural component of the skin, and act as an antioxidant in the skin, limiting damage by the sun.

Bleaches

B*leaches*, such as hydroquinone cream, can be applied to discolored areas about twice a day. Minor discolorations will remain lightened for a few months after treatment ends. Not as effective as AHA and slightly more expensive, bleaches are available both in prescription form and half-strength, nonprescription form. As with AHA, these may result in slight, temporary rashes in some individuals.

Injections

Injections of *collagen* (from cow hide), *fibrin* (gelatin made from pig tissue mixed with the patient's blood), or the patient's own *fat* (from abdomen or thigh) can smooth fine wrinkles and other minor pits and grooves. Effects can last for a few months to two years. Obviously, these treatments have no effect against discoloration, which becomes more of a problem in our 40s.

Younger-looking Hands

Other than the face, our hands and nails are probably the most noticeable parts of the body. If we remember to use sunscreen on the backs of our hands as well as other exposed skin, then that'll do a lot to protect the skin there from aging prematurely but despite our best skin care, so-called "liver spots" may begin to develop somewhere in our 30s, and become more noticeable in our 40s and 50s.

WHAT DO LIVER SPOTS HAVE TO DO WITH THE LIVER? "Liver spots" or "age spots" have nothing to do with the liver—they have more to do with genetics and exposure to the sun, which accelerates the process. They are actually superficial skin discolorations that are similar to freckles.

Most men can hope to find relief from liver spots within six months of applying Retin-A. There are milder options available as well, but Retin-A is the most popular.

OTHER TTHAN RETIN-A, WHAT ELSE CAN MAKE HANDS LOOK YOUNGER? One of these options involves removal of age spots by freezing them with liquid nitrogen and then applying a bleaching agent during the healing process. Mild skin peels can also be used but are more difficult to apply on the hands than on the face.

Another option is to treat fine wrinkles on the hands with injectable collagen, which plumps up the creases. But this is a temporary solution and needs to be repeated from time to time in order to maintain its effectiveness.

BEWARE ADVERTISING

Aside from dermabrasion, chemical peels, and Retin-A, it is important to understand that, other than alpha-hydroxy acids (AHA), no cosmetic product actually does anything other than keep the skin moist and make it look smoother while it is actually on the skin. Cosmetic advertisements would have us believe that certain ingredients have "antiaging" properties. Except for the sunscreen component offering protection from the aging effects of exposure to the sun, and AHAs, there is *absolutely no cosmetic* that functions in an anti-aging modality.

This needs to be stressed because of the intense efforts advertisers go to in order to confuse consumers. In the late 1980s the cosmetic industry clashed with the Food and Drug Administration to resolve how far advertisers could go in making claims about the antiaging properties of their products. The FDA finally decided in a letter to the cosmetic companies, that "all of the examples that you use to allege an effect within the epidermis as the basis for a temporary beneficial effect on wrinkles, lines or fine lines are unacceptable."

Yet, despite that decision, cosmetic ads continue to have us believe, through the very strategic use of language in ad copy, that their products do, indeed, slow down the aging process. Take, for example, the following statement in an ad by Lancôme:

> Based on the most recent findings to date, Lancôme research is now able to provide an age treatment product of inexpressive potency.

Doesn't that sound like more than mere moisturizer? Well, if it were, you can bet the FDA would demand it fall under their responsibility and insist on years of research before the product could be marketed.

What matters in the long run is not the brand of cosmetic you use, or the claims made by the advertisers, but rather the day-to-day care and consideration you give your skin. The cardinal priority, as I mentioned at the beginning of this chapter, is to minimize the aging effect of the sun. To look ten years younger, do that and keep your skin from drying out too much.

Beyond that, there remain the options of an occasional scrub and for a more intense approach, dermabrasion, chemical peel and, ultimately, Retin-A if your dermatologist agrees that it is appropriate for you.

Drinking 6–8 glasses of water each day, avoiding smoking, and not consuming too much alcohol are very important components of looking younger, as are proper nutrition and supplements.

I've taken a lot of time in this chapter to delve into the area of cosmetics because so many rely on false hopes promoted by advertisers. Other than moisturizers, you do *not* need cosmetics to look ten years younger.

THINGS YOU NEVER KNEW ABOUT SOAP

Now that Randy's beard had been removed and he had gotten rid of his wrinkles with a little help from his dermatologist, Randy was finding that his newly exposed skin was more sensitive to the soaps and lotions he was accustomed to using. "Doc," he said in his flippant manner, "can you give a 'short course' on soaps and lotions? I need to take care of this new 'baby skin' I've got." So here, for Randy and the rest of you, is the "short course."

Now that you've done your best to encourage younger skin, how do you best go about keeping that skin from drying out? We turn at this point to soaps and moisturizers, not merely to keep our skin from getting too dry but also to make it look and smell pleasant.

The Difference Between Soap and Detergent

The most common cosmetic is soap, the basic function of which is to allow water and dirt to combine, removing the resulting mixture from the skin. To be precise, soap is a mixture of sodium salts and various fatty acids of natural oils and fats, and comes in bars, granules, flakes or liquid form. The word itself probably comes from the Old English "sape," originally a reddish hair dye used by Germanic warriors to give a frightening appearance.

A detergent is a cleanser that is soapless, acidic rather than alkaline, and made from synthetics rather than natural animal fat. It may be preferable for those with very dry skin, but each man's skin has a unique response to various soaps or detergents.

To Moisturize Your Face, Use Lotions, Not Soap

In general, soaps will not add moisture to your skin, no matter what the ads proclaim. Even if the soaps contain moisturizers, these will be washed away along with the natural oils in your skin.

Those of you with thin, dry skin and light complexions may have more trouble with the drying effect of soap. So you may consider cleansing creams and lotions, but check with your dermatologist if these are problematic as well.

Everything You Always Wanted to Know About Soaps

Soaps, without which we couldn't survive as social beings in our culture, come in many forms and account for a great deal of confusion in the marketplace. This product is unregulated by the Food and Drug Administration because it isn't considered a cosmetic, unless it is advertised as such. Then the FDA does step in. So those soaps marketed as personal cleansing products (for example, anti-acne products) are regulated. Generally, if a soap is advertised as an *antimicrobial* or *anti-acne* product, it is regulated; otherwise, it isn't.

Here's an attempt to slug through some of the confusion about soaps. Although, technically speaking, a detergent is soap-free, and typically harsher on dry skin, that isn't always the case. Some detergents have added emollients making them even milder than the average soap, for example, Dove "soap" (really a detergent) as opposed to Ivory soap (an "old-fashioned" soap made by combining an alkali with fat and water).

The pH scale measures the degree of *acidity* (any value under 7) versus *alkalinity* (any value greater than 7). Under normal conditions, the skin is slightly acidic (pH = 4.5 to 6.5), being covered, on the surface, by dead skin cells, natural oils, and perspiration (all this typically referred to as the *acid mantle*).

The pH of a cleanser can be above 7 (basic) or below 7 (acidic). If a soap is very basic (or alkaline), it can have a somewhat irritating effect on dry skin. Soap is by nature alkaline. So if a nonalkaline cleanser is needed, a detergent "soap" becomes the product of choice. This, as I mentioned earlier, need not be harsh if the product contains soothing emollients.

Superfatted soaps are supposed to replace some of the oils they wash away by adding lanolin, oil, or cold cream to the soap itself, but there is a question among dermatologists as to whether or not this works. Theoretically, it is unlikely that a soap can "choose" to wash away some oils while depositing others onto the skin and leaving them intact.

FOUR ANTIAGING MOISTURIZING PRODUCTS FOR YOUR SKIN

An important consideration for keeping your skin ten years younger is what you put on your skin once it is cleaned up. I'm talking moisturizers—emollients, humectants, and other common, occasionally esoteric substances.

1. Petroleum Jelly—the Best and Cheapest

Emollients are basically softening agents, specially developed to protect the skin by relieving dryness, promoting a softer, smoother skin. The emollient essentially works by forming a barrier through which water will not pass. By far, the most effective, and least expensive emollient is petrolatum, known commercially as Vaseline. Tests at the University of Pennsylvania showed Vaseline to be the most effective moisturizer, lasting for two weeks after the application. An additional benefit of Vaseline is that it very rarely creates allergy problems. Unscented Vaseline is inert and will never cause allergy. Beware of "baby-fresh scent," however, if you *are* allergic.

2. Lanolin—the Most Natural

The next best emollient is lanolin, extracted from sheep wool, and an important ingredient in both expensive and inexpensive skin care products. In addition to preventing a loss of water from the skin, it helps soften the skin, being very close in composition to your own natural oil secretions. The only negative factor in lanolin is the possibility of creating acne-like problems if you're particularly prone to that. Since lanolin is so similar to your own natural oil secretions, it should come as no surprise that it can cause the same problems.

3. Mineral Oil—the Most Common

The third emollient, mineral oil, is the least effective of the three as a moisturizer. Yet it is the most common ingredient in skin care products.

4. Humectants—for Humid Environments

Humectants, usually *propylene glycol*, draw moisture from the air and then transfer it to the surface of the skin. How convenient! Unless the ambient air is very dry, and then the process reverses itself, drawing moisture from the skin. So humectants work best in a humid environment, and have the opposite effect in very dry situations.

   Why is dry skin a problem for some men and not others? And why sometimes and not other times?

What Causes Dry Skin

As mentioned earlier, as you get older, sweat glands and oil glands diminish in size and number, resulting in dryer skin. Beyond that, some men have naturally dryer skin than others; just born that way, if you will.

   As for circumstances resulting in dry skin:

1. using a very alkaline soap;

2. bathing too often, since this washes away the natural, protective oils of the skin;

3. dry air in winter, when the air is heated and dried as it circulates through the heating system (the average humidity in a sealed, heated building is 10 percent or less; relative humidity less than 30 percent begins to have a drying effect on the skin). Hence, the need for moisturizers, particularly if you bathe often with strongly alkaline soap in the wintertime.

The Difference Between Creams and Lotions

All you really need to restore moisture to your skin is water. The trick is to keep the water on your skin. That's where oil comes in. So a moisturizer is basically a mixture of oil and water. If there's more oil and less water, you have a cream or ointment; more water and less oil, you have a lotion. Creams are more effective but lotions are more popular, because they're less obvious in terms of appearance.

Sweat is nature's perfect moisturizer. So if Mother Nature is falling down on the job, such additives in moisturizers as urea and lactic acid (present in normal sweat) assist the moisturizer in its job.

Combining Moisturizers with Sunscreens

Ultimately, the best you can do to keep your skin ten years younger is a moisturizer that also protects it from the sun. Unless you live and work in a windowless environment, you're exposed to the sun on an ongoing basis, traveling to and from work, sitting near windows, doing your daily exercise, and so on. It would be very awkward and you'd run the risk of appearing to be a skin health fanatic if you were continually dabbing first moisturizer and then sunscreen on your face. Cosmetic manufacturers have not been asleep at the wheel. It was just a matter of time till they came up with products that combine both functions, and such products are currently on the market. There will be an increasing number of these dual-function products as we become more sophisticated about what it takes to keep looking ten years younger.

What to Use When

The most important thing is to adapt your skin-care habits to the climate you're in. In cold weather, you need a richer cream to protect and nourish your skin. In warm weather, you need a lighter lotion and a sunscreen.

AGE-PROOF YOUR SKIN WITH VITAMINS

Randy was quite happy with his new skin and his new knowledge of caring for it. Now he wanted to know how best to feed his new skin. So my talk with Randy turned to vitamins.

We've already covered the basics in earlier chapters. The main additional information relates to vitamin A (also known as retinol), because of its association with Retin-A (not the same, but definitely in the same chemical family); vitamin E (tocopherol) because of research attributing to it a helpful function in dealing with ultraviolet light; and vitamin C because of its ability, along with bioflavinoids, to reduce collagen breakdown.

Vitamin A

Vitamin A, or its precursor, beta carotene, found in yellow and green vegetables, is essential to the good health of skin cells. Without it, skin becomes dry and scaly, looking ten years older rather than how we'd like it.

Retinoids

In the last few years, retinoids, a new class of drugs related to vitamin A, have been developed and marketed to help keep your skin looking years younger. Topical applications of Retin-A and certain oral drugs are available from dermatologists to help you keep your skin looking better and younger.

Vitamin E

Vitamin E is purported to help keep the skin healthy. A good source is vegetable oils. One interesting facet of this vitamin is that it can be applied directly to the skin with positive effect and consequently is often found as a component of skin creams and lotions.

Vitamin C

Vitamin C has been discussed at length in Chapter 6. It provides many benefits, one of the primary ones being the maintenance of good health and the structural integrity of your blood vessels. Since the skin is so sensitive (at least in appearance) to its blood supply, then it stands to reason that vitamin C is essential to looking younger.

The B Vitamins

The B vitamins are also essential to good skin care. The skin disease, pellagra, is an essential symptom of niacin deficiency. This is rarely seen though, except in chronic alcoholics with extremely poor nutrition habits.

In the absence of other B vitamins, a man's skin becomes red and begins to peel, dry cracks appear at the corners of the mouth, and a scaly rash develops on the face. Deficiency of B_{12} can result in skin changes such as extreme pallor, so a B-complex vitamin is strongly encouraged along with your daily vitamin/mineral regimen.

Your skin, like the rest of your body, needs a balanced, healthy supply of nutrients. Given the balanced food supply recommended in the Ryback Food Plan, you need not worry about lack of nutrients. Since fried foods and those rich in fat are strongly discouraged, your skin should be receiving a healthy balance of nutrients.

Look Young, Not Foolish

I want to point out that, except for vitamin A-related Retin-A and possibly vitamin E, all other nutrients applied directly to the skin have no nutritional or any other direct effect on the skin except for the moisturizing effect of their oils. Avocado extracts and mink oil essences absolutely do not "feed" the skin except to keep it moist. So if you're going to spend money on vitamins for your skin, spend it on the ones you put in your mouth rather than around it. You want to keep looking young, though not necessarily foolish.

WHY CIGARETTES AND EXCESSIVE ALCOHOL MAKE YOU LOOK OLD

What you do *not* want to put in your mouth, if you're to keep your skin looking years younger, are cigarette smoke and too much alcohol.

Remember W. C. Fields' claim to fame? His red, bulbous nose—the facial signature of the inveterate alcoholic. This condition, known medically as *rosacea*, results from the dilation of blood vessels, often aggravated by excessive drinking. Although alcohol is not the only factor contributing to this condition, it is one we have direct control over if we choose to.

Smoking—Bad for Skin and Teeth

Smoking not only keeps you from living ten years longer, it keeps you from looking ten years younger as well. It's well known that smoking causes wrinkling and drying of skin around the mouth, by damaging the outer "barrier" layer of skin. In addition to prematurely wrinkling the facial skin, smoking also yellows the teeth and fingernails. Resins and tar from smoking tobacco build up on the teeth, making plaque and tartar more difficult to remove. Smoking, all told, is a poor choice if you're intent on looking ten years younger.

Smoking, as I'll discuss in the next chapter, allows for carbon monoxide to replace the oxygen in the blood and otherwise to narrow the blood vessels, resulting in decreased oxygen flow to the growing skin cells. This is most notable in the premature wrinkling of the skin. Simply put, to look ten years younger, don't smoke, and drink moderately, if at all.

Inexpensive Cosmetic Surgery for Your Eyes

Plastic surgery is not something to be entered into lightly (or inexpensively) but, for those who choose it, a face lift can certainly counter the aging effects that become more noticeable in the 40s.

One alternative to conventional surgery is a new micro-liposuction procedure. This relatively inexpensive procedure involves making a small incision at the site of a scar-hiding wrinkle in the corner of the eye, and vacuuming out the undesirable accumulations of fatty tissue just under the eye. This results in a more youthful look without the expense of regular surgery.

YOUR HAIR AS YOU AGE

As if he hadn't done enough to capture the woman of his dreams, Randy was now concerned that his balding pate might drive her away. Randy was not yet bald by any means, but at the same time it was clear that his hairline *was* receding. If he didn't take action soon, not only would he lose his apparent hair, but he'd run out of time to get an heir apparent with the wife for whom he was searching. What to do about baldness was Randy's most current concern.

It's sometimes frightening to see so much hair being lost when we shampoo. I thought I was going bald when I was a teenager because of this, but it's quite natural to see a lot of hair going down the drain when we wash. People differ greatly on this, but unless we see our hair thinning and receding on our scalp, slight hair loss in itself is not a worrisome process, just the normal process of turnover. If you continue to eat your veggies and take your vitamin and mineral supplements, you're feeding your hair properly. Crash diets, which I strongly discourage, can sometimes result in a greater than usual loss of hair.

Yet, despite healthy diet and proper hair grooming, some men begin to lose their hair at relatively young ages. Why do men become bald? It is a question that has intrigued us for a long time.

Starting in our early adulthood, it's normal to lose one percent of the hair on our heads. For most of us, serious hair loss doesn't become a problem until we get to our 50s. But for about 50 million men in the U.S., *pattern baldness*, known scientifically as *androgenetic alopecia*, becomes a severe problem at a younger age. All we know is that such men appear to have a genetic predisposition to the presence of male hormones, or androgens.

For men, balding is localized, occurring in the front, in the center, or on the crown of the head. Sometimes it's a combination of the three, but it's usually most visibly noticeable as a receding hair line.

WHAT TO DO ABOUT BALDING

Although a completely bald head is a fashion statement in itself (Yul Brynner, Telly Savalas, Patrick Stewart, an increasing number of athletes), most men become gravely concerned about a noticeably receding hairline or a visible balding spot at the crown of the head. Whether or not you choose the bald look and enjoy the unique attention it brings you is a personal choice. A goodly number of attractive, virile-looking men enjoy such a fashionable look. For those who choose the hairy alternative and notice the beginnings of "wavy" hair (in other words, hair "waving" good-bye), here's what to do. . . .

There are basically three approaches to conquer the balding process:

1. Drugs and Electricity

The use of electricity is somewhat in dispute, but to the extent that it works, it does so by "waking up" quiescent follicles through electrical stimulation. The balding man sits beneath a hairdryer-like hood for 12 minutes while his scalp is bathed in a low-level electrical field. A dermatologist from the University of British Columbia found a two-thirds increase in hair counts in his research subjects. This process was first developed by the Vancouver company, Current Technology.

The use of drugs is quite popular with balding men. The most common of these is *Rogaine* (*minoxidil*), approved for the Upjohn Co. by the FDA in 1988. About two thirds of those who use it find that it prevents further hair loss, and about one third find that it actually causes significant regrowth of hair. It's fairly expensive, though, costing upward of $60 a month for 6 months. The commercial success of Rogaine ($143 million in annual worldwide sales) has prompted more research in this area.

A somewhat new kid on the block is Merck's prescription drug, *Proscar* (*finasteride*), first developed to treat prostate gland enlargement in men, but found to counteract baldness as well. Proscar works by preventing the formation of *androgen*, which is involved in the demise of scalp follicles. Other baldness-fighting drugs currently being researched are *Tricomin* which works by incorporating protein

into the hair shaft; and *aromatase*, which works by encouraging follic-
ular activity in the scalp. Aromatase is an enzyme which men appear
to lack.

Drugs and electricity are approaches that both men and women
can use. The next two approaches are much more likely to be used by
men.

2. Scalp Reduction

In this approach, a flap of hair-bearing scalp is moved from the side
of the head to the top of the head. The barren scalp is surgically
removed and the healthy flap is then stretched over this new area.
The healthy hair flaps are genetically programmed to last a lifetime,
unlike the hair on the top of these individuals' heads. This procedure
is called scalp reduction. The downside of this procedure is its cost,
being upwards of $15,000.

3. Micrografting

This involves placing single hair grafts from the sides and back of the
scalp onto the balding area. The surgical grafts are done in a random,
feathering pattern to create a natural hairline, rather than lining up
larger grafts in unnatural, straight lines. This procedure has improved
over the past few years, avoiding the older, "tufted" look, in essence
creating a "no hairline" hairline. This procedure requires about four
visits six to eight weeks apart, costing somewhere in the neighborhood of $2,000 per session, for a grand total of about $8,000 to
$10,000. Each "stab wound" is about $1\frac{1}{4}$ millimeters wide, contain-
ing a maximum of 3 hairs. Since the grafts are so tiny, healing occurs
quickly and the patient can go back to work the day after each surgical session.

COLORING AWAY THE GRAY

Randy's primary reason for cutting off his beard was that it was turning gray. So he cut it off. But now the hair on his head—once he had
taken care of the balding issue—was, of course, beginning to turn

gray as well. Still on the hunt for his dream woman, Randy couldn't afford to let grayness slow his pursuit. Randy was not alone in his concern with the older look of graying hair.

A major consideration for hair in the endeavor to look ten years younger is the graying process which can start in the 30s for many men. Of course, highlighting and semipermanent color are the best covers for early gray. If you're new to the graying process, then the best products for you to explore might be Clairol's Lasting Color by Loving Care and L'Oreal's Casting Tone-on-Tone. Both of these sink into the hair shaft and change color by chemical reaction, yet they're less harmful than permanent color can be. Instead of leaving obvious signs of demarcation as time goes by, the color simply fades away, and the natural nuances of the original colors return gradually. The effect lasts up to 20 shampoos or 6 weeks (whichever comes first); the cost is about $7 to $8 per bottle.

Although men can use these products just as easily as women, they can choose those with marketing focused directly at them. Clairol offers five shades of Men's Choice and Grecian Formula offers Just For Men, a 5-minute gray-covering treatment which comes in several shades.

MAINTAINING YOUR HAIR'S YOUTHFUL SHINE

As we mature into our 40s, hair tends to shrink in diameter, making it finer and more fragile, while becoming more limp. There are many shampoos and conditioners which take into account the changing disposition of hair. As we enter middle age, our scalps tend to become drier, as our oil glands become less active. Choose shampoos geared for dry hair. Also, take it easy with the hair dryer. Try using it on a lower setting and for less time. During the winter, hot-oil treatments may help as well.

HOW TO KEEP YOUNGER-LOOKING TEETH

Just as visible as the skin is the changing state of our teeth as we get older. Even in our 30s, teeth may begin to discolor, both because of the accumulated effect of food stains (not to mention tobacco stains) and because of the thinning of tooth enamel, revealing the yellow dentin from under the enamel. As we get into our 40s, teeth may begin to move around slightly, creating crookedness, crowding, or gaps. By now some of the fillings we've had since younger years may begin to wear around the edges. For those of us in our 40s, our gums may begin to recede due to gum disease, which requires professional attention. Our teeth continue to weaken for a variety of reasons, so that, by our 50s, our teeth become more brittle and susceptible to breakage when suddenly confronted with a cherry pit or other unexpected hard object.

How to Keep Your Gums from Receding

Well, sink your teeth into this advice for looking ten years younger. First of all, twice-a-year visits to your dentist for a cleaning and once-over inspection are a must, no matter what your age. Keeping your teeth free of tartar or plaque will help keep your gums strong and supple, delaying the onset of gum recession. Another must, regardless of age, is proper brushing and flossing. Check with your dentist for the proper technique. Improper brushing can cause your gum line to start receding prematurely. It's something you'll be doing on a daily basis, and doing it right takes no more energy, yet might make all the difference.

Contouring and Veneers

While you're at your dentist, ask him to discuss the possibility of contouring or shaping your teeth to improve your appearance. It may just be a matter of polishing the edges of a couple or so teeth to make their alignment more attractive when you smile. It'll only take a few extra seconds of your dentist's time, if indeed he thinks it necessary. While you're at it, you might ask your dentist about dealing with discoloration through a number of options—*bleaching, bonding,* or *porcelain veneers*. Most actors have relied on at least one of these so that their teeth look gleaming white in those revealing close-up photos. Even the gaps that might occur in your 40s and 50s can sometimes be improved by judicious use of veneers. And of course veneers can sometimes avoid tooth replacement if you should happen to chip a tooth that becomes more brittle as you get into your 50s and 60s.

PUTTING IT ALL TOGETHER

I'll say it one more time. Staying out of the sun or protecting the skin with sunscreen is the most important thing you can do. "Suffice it to say," agrees dermatologist Tom Sternberg, "the sun is the greatest single factor in premature aging of the skin."

Beyond that, proper nutrition, along with water, vitamins, and minerals, is very important. Your skin, reports Dr. Richard Walzer, "is one of the first organs to reflect a deficiency or excess of vitamins in the body."

So looking ten years younger isn't that complicated. This chapter only underscores the importance of the previous chapters. Vitamins, minerals, proper nutrition, avoidance of smoking, and maintaining a strong cardiovascular system through exercise for healthy circulation to the skin, are all important.

All cosmetics can do is keep your skin moist and protect it from the sun (if they contain sunscreen). Hopefully, this chapter has made you an educated consumer of soaps and cosmetics. And it has made you somewhat more aware of what your dermatologist can do to help you create younger-looking skin.

And if you're still skeptical about looking ten years younger, look at it this way: Without following the suggestions in the previous chapters and particularly in this one, you're sure to look older than your chronological age. So even if you start now to follow these recommendations, you'll stop the aggravating effects of poor nutrition, smoking, and sun on the aging of your skin. Compared to all others who eat poorly, smoke, and expose themselves to harmful sun rays, you *will* look ten years younger. For the rest of your life!

— SIDEBAR I —

"SOAP TRANQUILIZERS" FOR YOUTHFUL SKIN

One recent and interesting use of soap deserves mention. Scientists at the Memorial Sloan-Kettering's Psychiatry Service have experimented with the tranquilizing effects of a vanilla-like scent called *heliotropin* on patients undergoing the often claustrophobia-inducing magnetic resonance imaging test (MRI). Results indicated that those patients exposed to the fragrance were 63 percent less anxious than those not exposed to this soothing aroma. What if we could attach such an aroma to everyday soap? Could we become both clean *and* relaxed in one application?

Well, guess what! Scientists at Yale's Psychophysical Center have explored the use of lavender as a calming fragrance. So any lavender soap (for example, Lavender Glycerine Soap from Thymes Ltd.) can soothe our minds while it soothes the skin on our faces.

— SIDEBAR II —

SLEEPING FOR YOUNGER-LOOKING SKIN

To look ten years younger, give yourself enough sleep time. During sleep, a number of specific skin growth factors are released along with human growth hormone. These hormones may speed up the production of collagen, the protein that's responsible for elasticity and support of the skin, encouraging a more youthful rate of exfoliation.

— SIDEBAR III —

BUYING THE MOST EFFECTIVE SUNSCREEN

There are as many as 40 pathological skin conditions related to sun exposure, ranging from skin eruptions and sunburn to skin cancer. Sunscreen products continue to improve. A broad-spectrum product is always best, covering the A, B, and C forms of ultraviolet rays. Currently under study is a new product, *Prozone,* which includes a 1 percent concentration of the natural skin pigment melanin, producing a highly effective broad-spectrum sunscreen. Melanin has a natural antiaging effect on the skin (due to its antioxidant properties) and we'll probably be seeing more of this substance in skin-care products as time rolls by.

Products with a high SPF have both a greater number of screening chemicals as well as more of each one. Sunscreens come in many forms these days: lotions, thicker creams, gels, watery liquids that have alcohol bases, and aerosol sprays. A few of the waterproof sunscreens that perform well also have a sweet odor, if you enjoy that. Sun-screens with an alcohol base are better for those with oily skin. The other forms are preferable for those with dry skin. Alcohol-based screens are usually clear and are often described as having a "cool alcohol formula," while the others are creams and look it, and use words like "cream" or "oil."

— SIDEBAR IV —

How to Keep Younger Teeth

Age 30: Teeth may begin to discolor.
Tooth enamel thins.

Age 40: Teeth may move slightly, causing crookedness or gaps.
Gums may begin to recede.
Old fillings begin to deteriorate.

Age 50: Teeth become more brittle and susceptible to breaking.

What to do:

1. Proper brushing and flossing.
2. Twice-a-year visits to your dentist for inspection and cleaning.
3. Consider bleaching, bonding, or porcelain veneers.
4. Also, consider contouring or shaping of teeth.

— SIDEBAR V —

How to Keep Younger Hair

Graying of hair can start as early as the 30s, or may occur very late in life. What to do:

1. If you're new to the graying process, try highlighting your hair with henna or vegetable dyes that accent the natural color of your hair.
2. As a more advanced step, try semipermanent color products such as Clairol's Men's Choice and Grecian Formula's Just for Men.
3. If you choose permanent coloring, you commit yourself to retouching sessions on a monthly basis as roots need attention as they grow out.

Into the 40s, hair tends to become thinner, more fragile and limper. The scalp becomes drier. What to do:

1. Keep your hair from becoming even drier from overexposure to the sun.
2. Keep your hair healthy from within by sticking with the vitamin regimen recommended in the chapter on supplements.
3. Consider changing your hairstyle to shorter, bolder cuts.
4. Choose your shampoos and conditioners with more care. Experiment until you find products that leave you happy.
5. Heat is an enemy to hair. Minimize the use of blow dryers.
6. During cold weather, treat yourself to hot-oil treatments.

— SIDEBAR VI —

How to Keep Younger Skin

Age 30: As cell turnover begins to slow down, skin may begin to appear somewhat duller.

1. Avoid overexposure to the sun.
2. Use broad-spectrum sunscreens such as Photoplex by Herbert Labs or Shade UVAGuard by Schering-Plough.
3. Consider superficial chemical peels.

Age 40: Skin may begin to show discoloring or moles. It also thins out slightly. Crow's feet may begin to develop around the eyes.

1. Talk with your dermatologist about using Retin-A.
2. While you're at it, discuss the benefits of facial scrubs and dermabrasion.

Age 50: Wrinkling becomes more prominent.

1. Time to consider deep chemical peels.
2. Alpha-hydroxy acids (AHA) in cream and lotion form can speed up the rate of exfoliation.

Age 60: Fat pockets may form under eyes. Facial skin becomes slack. Wrinkling increases.

1. New technologies in plastic surgery are worth considering.
2. Bleaches can be applied to discolored areas.
3. Injections of collagen, fibrin, or your own fat can reclaim your original, youthful contour.

Age 70: Your true character is now on display for the world to enjoy.

1. Hopefully, you're living your life with integrity, so that you're proud of your character showing on your face.

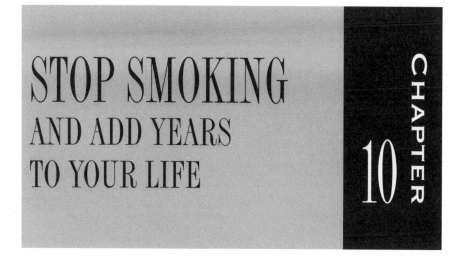

STOP SMOKING
AND ADD YEARS
TO YOUR LIFE

In the prime of his life, at the age of 38, Dr. Sigmund Freud was frightened by the irregular heartbeats he felt in his chest. He consulted his own physician, and was advised to give up his smoking habit. This great healer of the human psyche did so, of course, and had this to say about it:

> There were tolerable days. . . Then came suddenly a severe affectation of the heart, worse than I ever had when smoking. . . And with it an oppression of mood in which images of dying and farewell scenes replaced the more usual fantasies . . . It is annoying for a doctor who has to be concerned all day long with neurosis, not to know whether he is suffering from a justifiable or hypochondriacal depression. (From "The Life and Works of Sigmund Freud," by Ernest Jones, N.Y.: Basic Books, Vol. I, pp. 309–310.)

And as you might suspect, Dr. Freud yielded to his human frailties and succumbed to smoking once again—twenty cigars a day. And continued, except for one 14-month abstention, for the rest of his life, despite the fact that he admitted that it interfered with his studies.

By age 67, Freud developed cancer in his mouth and jaw. Thirty-three operations later, he continued to smoke until he actually lost his jaw. The artificial jaw caused him much pain and made it very difficult for him to swallow. He remained addicted to smoking right up to his cancer-induced death.

Freud was undeniably a brilliant individual. He mastered the workings of the human mind. He was skilled at hypnosis. He was well trained in medicine and biology. Yet this physician was not able to heal his own smoking addiction. He failed, and did not learn from his own failings in this particular area of behavior.

Today, there is a difference, thanks in large part to a change in the public's perception of smoking. In 1954, Eva Cooper sued the R.J. Reynolds Tobacco Co. for contributing to her husband's death due to cancer. The court ruled that there was insufficient evidence to prove that the Camels her husband smoked caused his illness. But those who valued their health fought back. By 1983, San Francisco passed the country's first strong workplace antismoking ordinance.

In 1988, smoking was banned on domestic flights of less than 2 hours. By 1994, the banner against smoking was raised when the U.S. Surgeon General spoke up for government regulation of cigarettes. The tide was finally beginning to turn.

The FDA was considering reclassifying tobacco as a drug. The Labor Department proposed prohibiting smoking in all indoor workplaces. A class-action lawsuit was filed in New Orleans against six tobacco companies for deceiving the public.

Today a body of knowledge exists that allows us to learn from our failings. This body of knowledge informs us of the specific chemistry of the biological damage of smoking: the statistics that link smoking to cancer, emphysema, heart disease, cholesterol build-up; the biological and psychological consequences of quitting once you're addicted; and, finally, what methods work best, which "quitting technologies" have the best track record. In this chapter, we'll take a look at all of this. So that if you fail, you can learn from your failure and start again. And again. All the way to ultimate success and added years of life.

PERSISTENCE LEADS TO SUCCESS

The bad news is that of all who are successful at quitting, as many as 80 percent will suffer relapses. The good news is that those who learn from their first fall from grace will be more successful the next time around. The great news is that, for those men who persist, recognizing failure as a learning path to greater chances of success the next time around, success is virtually guaranteed. Unfortunately, Freud didn't know this. Had he had this information available, I'm certain he would have avoided the excruciating pain of jaw cancer which afflicted his final years. He might even have lived longer.

The process of quitting smoking is a circular path—actually more like a circular coil. The ultimate goal—being smoke-free—is in the center. We start at the outer edge and work our way to the center. It takes four steps to go around the circle once. Every time we complete a revolution we get closer to the center—the goal. If you're among the lucky 20 percent of men who can do it first time around, then there's only one coil in your circle. If it takes you five falls from grace, then there are five coils in your circle.

The four steps to complete each revolution are as follows:

Denial ➤ Conflict ➤ Action ➤ Change

Overcome Your Denial

Half the struggle of quitting smoking, then, is overcoming the denial that smoking is a form of systematic suicide and getting through the conflict of being responsible for making your life both shorter as well as miserable except for the immediate gratification of smoking.

Making the Decision—the Key to Success

When a smoker comes to my office to discuss quitting, he's already into the second step, *Conflict*. Thank goodness, I don't have to deal with his *Denial*. That's already been taken care of by his spouse, his family doctor, or certain excruciating pains in his chest. Increasingly, I'm happy to add, the workplace is becoming more involved in that process of encouraging smoke-free environments. So he comes into my office and asks: "Dr. Ryback, can you make me quit smoking?"

"No!" I retort adamantly. "I refuse to treat you unless *you* have made a clear and definite decision to quit. Then I'll do what I can to help you. And only then!" If he was still in *Conflict* when he sat down, by the time he arises from that chair, he's made a decision one way or another. Almost always, the decision is to quit. But it's *his* decision, not mine. And that, my dear reader, is the key to this chapter.

If you have not made a clear decision to quit, then I'll bet a hundred dollars to a dozen doughnuts (or whole wheat bagels) that you will not be successful, no matter what techniques you use, from hypnosis to having your ears stapled. On the other hand, if you've made a clear and honest decision to quit, then I'll have my bagels with fat-free cream cheese, thank you.

Commitment to Change

So now we begin, as the psychiatrist says at the end of "Portnoy's Complaint." The *Action* stage begins with commitment. Once you have commitment, success is merely the follow-through. It's a matter of going through the steps of whatever technology you choose. And that technology must be integrated with some lifestyle *Change*, the fourth step of the cycle.

If at First You Don't Succeed

For most men who go through these four steps to success and then, for whatever reason, fail, there is a whole new cycle of *Denial, Conflict, Action,* and *Change*. It isn't easy. But with persistence, you will succeed. Each cycle gets easier—the coils get smaller as you approach the center, and you learn from each cycle. And you progress—and ultimately succeed.

First of all, let's define smoking addiction. According to the *Diagnostic and Statistical Manual of Mental Disorders* which psychiatrists and psychologists use, the diagnostic criteria for tobacco withdrawal are as follows:

A. Use of tobacco for at least several weeks at a level equivalent to more than ten cigarettes per day, with each cigarette containing at least 0.5 mg of nicotine.

B. Abrupt cessation of or reduction in tobacco use, followed within 24 hours by at least four of the following:

1. craving for tobacco

2. irritability

3. anxiety

4. difficulty in concentrating

5. restlessness

6. headache

7. drowsiness

8. gastrointestinal disturbances

Sound familiar? Isn't it nice to have a label put to it? Doesn't feel so lonely any more, does it?

FOUR WAYS THAT SMOKING WILL KILL YOU

1. Cigarette "Tar"

Well, what causes all that discomfort, listed so neatly from 1 to 8? Unfortunately, the answer is neither neat nor simple. The "tar" in cigarette smoke is comprised of several thousand chemicals, including *acids, glycol, aldehydes, ketones,* as well as such corrosive and poisonous gases as *hydrogen cyanide* and *carbon monoxide.*

2. Carbon Monoxide Poison

Carbon monoxide comprises a relatively large 4 percent of the smoke and, once it enters the lungs, bullies its way into the red blood cells, pushing aside the oxygen that would otherwise be there. This substance deprives the heart and other tissues of essential oxygen and promotes cholesterol deposits in the arteries.

3. Nicotine

Nicotine itself is a poison that initially stimulates the brain and central nervous system, but subsequently has a depressant effect on it.

That's precisely why cigarettes act both as a stimulant and as a relaxant. The initial reaction is that of a picker-upper but after a few minutes, becomes quite relaxing. It is this paradoxical effect that makes smoking so desirable. It's good for what ails you, in the sense that it will stimulate you if you're bored and listless; it will relax you if you're anxious and stressed. What a great substance! If only it didn't rob you of years of life in the process.

4. One Hundred Fifty Thousand Yearly Deaths Reported

If that weren't bad enough, many of the components of cigarette smoke are carcinogenic. It has been argued that 30 percent of all cancer deaths can be attributed to smoking, particularly cancers of the lung, larynx, mouth, and esophagus. It also contributes to cancers of the bladder, pancreas, and kidney.

Of all the cancers, the most fatal are those occurring in the lungs and pancreas. The American Cancer Society informs us that about 150,000 persons lose their lives each year because of tobacco smoking.

PROOF THAT SMOKING KILLS. In 1951, the British Medical Association sent a questionnaire on smoking habits to over 34,000 of its members. For the twenty years following, records were kept on changes in smoking habits and the causes of all deaths.

For these British doctors, the risk of dying of a heart attack before age 45 was *fifteen* times greater for heavy smokers than for nonsmokers. For lung cancers, respiratory diseases, and strokes, the risk of death was at least *three* times as high in smokers as in nonsmokers. A whole host of other types of cancer and various diseases were just slightly correlated with smoking. Overall, you can see that the case against smoking is made quite strong by this extensive study, extensive both in terms of number of subjects and time span.

BREATHE EASIER AND LIVE LONGER: PREVENTING HEART AND LUNG DISEASE

Lung cancer starts off very slowly. There are few symptoms until the cancer is very advanced. What we call "cigarette cough" has nothing to do with cancer itself. It is merely the lungs trying to get rid of the accumulated smoke deposits. It appears the self-cleaning lining of the airways is knocked unconscious or disabled by the smoke. The cilia, tiny hair-like structures which sweep the airways clean, recover overnight and try to make a clean sweep of things in the morning before they're once again knocked out by the next day's smoke. It is their feeble attempt at a clean sweep that produces "cigarette cough."

In Chapter Eight, we explored the effect of poor nutrition on atherosclerosis, the build-up of cholesterol in the arteries. Smoking is a heavy contributor to this as well. Dr. Ronald Selvester studied the coronary angiograms of 104 heart disease patients in California. Of these, 60 did not smoke and the remaining 44 continued to smoke throughout the study. After 18 months of diet and exercise, the patients were once again tested. The results showed a significant worsening of coronary artery disease in 60 percent of the vessels of the smokers, compared to only 32 percent of the vessels of the nonsmokers—almost twice as much. Apparently, smoking appears to contribute significantly to the heart-cholesterol problem.

Smoking Less—Living More

There is a well-known ongoing debate between the tobacco industry and health-care advocates on the smoking/lung cancer correlation. The industry claims, to this very day, that there is no proof of smoking leading to lung cancer. Well, technically and legally, they're right. Proof would entail controlling the smoking habits of a group of individuals, rather than letting them choose for themselves. That, of course, is entirely unethical. So the industry will go on claiming there is no proof, and they're technically correct.

The Longer You Smoke, the Faster You Die

But, according to the World Health Organization, death rates are uniformly higher among smokers than among nonsmokers of both sexes. Among smokers, the death rates from all causes increase with the number of cigarettes smoked per day, the number of years the smoker has smoked, and the earlier the age at which smoking started.

Add Seven Years to Your Life

So how much will smoking cessation contribute to your new-found, more becoming, and more comfortable ten years? Well, if we look at statistical averages, it appears that nonsmokers start dying off at age 72 while smokers start doing so at age 65. That is, the longevity curves for nonsmokers starts declining at 72, and for smokers at 65. By age 80, about 60 percent of nonsmokers are still alive, compared to only 30 percent of smokers.

Another point of view: For those between the ages of 45 and 64, the death rate due to lung cancer is four times as great for smokers as compared to nonsmokers. For those from 65 to 79, that rate is nine times higher for the smokers.

Well, tobacco industry, put that in your pipe and smoke it! How 'bout those data? But some people will never be convinced, including those in the Denial stage. They may point out, "My uncle smoked heavily all his life and never got cancer." For that matter, look at George Burns, with his omnipresent cigar, making jokes about chasing women in his nineties (alive and well at the time of this writing). The overall picture is quite clear, though: Cigarette smokers die younger than nonsmokers.

IT'S NEVER TOO LATE TO QUIT

Stopping smoking will have a very direct effect on keeping your heart healthy, especially in the advanced years. A study of over 2,500 people from 65 to 74 years of age showed that older cigarette smokers had a risk of heart disease death over 50 percent higher than that of nonsmokers and exsmokers. Even among those who had smoked for many years, quitting smoking brought heart disease risks down to nonsmoking levels within one to five years.

So if you've been smoking for years, is it too late to quit? *Absolutely not!* As long as cancer has not yet started, the effects of smoking are definitely reversible. According to the American Cancer Society, here's what happens once you quit:

1. Within a few days mucus in your airways breaks up and clears out of your lungs.

2. Within a few weeks, circulation improves and you will be able to smell and taste more.

3. Within a year, your risk of lung cancer begins to decrease.

In case there's any doubt about the challenge to quitting smoking, let me share this very impressive piece of writing with you, by an expert on smoking.

Why Quitting Is So Painful

First of all, quitting is not easy. According to Walter Ross, a writer on smoking for over 15 years:

> When smokers first quit smoking, their heart rate slows, their blood pressure rises, brain waves register changes. In heavily-ddicted smokers, temperature drops; in less-addicted smokers, it rises. All quitters do less well in coordination tests, including driving, than they did when they were smoking. Mouth ulcers are common in quitters. There are sometimes more bizarre effects.

Larry, a 42-year-old schoolteacher of math and algebra, was smoking about a pack and a half a day. He had two children, 5 and 7, and Larry began to worry not only about setting a poor example, but also about the effect of passive smoke on them. His wife smoked, but unlike Larry, never in the house or in front of the children. Larry had good motivation to stop.

Larry tried time and again, once even using the nicotine patch. When he came to my office, he was desperate. I was his last-ditch effort. (Larry's story continues on p. 281.)

How to Discover the Years You'll Gain

In order to decide to quit, you need all the motivation you can get. How about living longer? We've already discussed the statistical data demonstrating a seven-year addition to your lifespan just by not smoking. To be precise, however, it really depends on your age when you quit. That seven-year difference applies to the contrast between those who smoke and those who have not smoked since at least age 35. If you quit before age 40, you can add five years to your life. If you quit by age 50, you can add three years. If you've been smoking up to the age of 70 and quit then, you can still benefit by one additional year of life. Incidentally, this doesn't mean that if you're 70 and quit smoking, you'll live to 71. No! It means that if you quit smoking at that age, you'll live one year longer than you otherwise would, most probably somewhere in your eighties or nineties, especially if you follow my suggestions in this book.

Are You Addicted?

First of all, let's find out if you're really addicted to smoking. You're clearly addicted if:

1. You light up within 30 minutes of awakening and that's your most satisfying cigarette of the day.

2. You smoke more than 25 high-nicotine cigarettes a day.

3. You smoke more before noon than during the rest of the day.

4. It's almost impossible to heed "no smoking" signs, as in restaurants and theaters.

If these are true for you, then it's going to be particularly rough to quit. The good news is, you *can* do it. But you'll have to go cold-turkey. No weaning process for you. If you're not addicted, there are some others ways to approach quitting. To find out what motivates you to smoke, take a few minutes to take the test on the following page, developed by the National Institutes of Health.

5 = Always   2 = Seldom
4 = Usually   1 = Never
3 = Sometimes

A.	I smoke cigarettes to keep myself from slowing down.	5 4 3 2 1
B.	Handling and touching a cigarette is part of enjoying smoking.	5 4 3 2 1
C.	I feel pleasant and relaxed when I smoke.	5 4 3 2 1
D.	I light up when I feel tense or mad about something.	5 4 3 2 1
E.	When I run out of cigarettes, I can hardly stand it until I get more.	5 4 3 2 1
F.	I smoke automatically; I am not always aware when I am smoking.	5 4 3 2 1
G.	Smoking helps me feel stimulated, turned on, creative.	5 4 3 2 1
H.	Part of my enjoyment comes in the steps I take to light up.	5 4 3 2 1
I.	For me, cigarettes are simply pleasurable.	5 4 3 2 1
J.	I light up when I feel upset or uncomfortable about something.	5 4 3 2 1
K.	I am quite aware of it when I am not smoking a cigarette.	5 4 3 2 1
L.	I may light up not realizing that I still have a cigarette in the ashtray.	5 4 3 2 1
M.	I smoke because cigarettes give me a "lift."	5 4 3 2 1
N.	Part of the pleasure of smoking is watching the smoke as I exhale.	5 4 3 2 1
O.	I want a cigarette most when I am relaxed and comfortable.	5 4 3 2 1
P.	I smoke when I am blue or want to take my mind off my worries.	5 4 3 2 1
Q.	I get "hungry" for a cigarette when I have not smoked for a while.	5 4 3 2 1
R.	I often find a cigarette in my mouth and don't remember putting it there.	5 4 3 2 1

For each category below, a score of 11 or more is high, 8 to 10 is medium, and 7 or less is low.

STIMULATION CATEGORY. Total your answers to A, G, and M. If the total is more than 9, you rely on cigarettes to stimulate and enliven you, to help you work, organize, or be creative. You are a good candidate for a substitute of another kind of "high"; five minutes of exercise in your office, a brisk walk.

TACTILE CATEGORY. Total your answers to B, H, and N. If the total is 9 or above, an important aspect of your smoking is the feel of it. Try substituting a pen or pencil, doodling, or occupying yourself with a small toy. You may want to squeeze a tennis ball or handgrip exerciser, or even hold a plastic cigarette.

PLEASURE CATEGORY. Total your answers to C, I, and O. A high score suggests that you are one of the people for whom cigarettes provide some real pleasure. If this is you, you are a particularly good candidate to stop because you can substitute other pleasurable outlets—reasonable eating, social, sports, or physical activities—for smoking.

TENSION CATEGORY. Total your answers to D, J, and P. Those who score high here use tobacco as a crutch, to reduce negative feelings, relieve problems, much like a tranquilizer. You are likely to find it easy to quit when things are going well, but staying off is harder in bad times. For you, the key is to find other activities that also work to reduce negative feelings: dancing, meditation, yoga, sports or exercise, meals, or social activities work for many such smokers.

ADDICTION CATEGORY. Total your answers to E, K, and Q. Quitting is hard for those who score high in this group because you are probably psychologically addicted and crave cigarettes. You aren't likely to succeed by tapering off gradually. Instead, try smoking more than usual for a day or two, until the craving dulls, then drop it cold turkey, and *isolate yourself* from cigarettes for a long period. There is good news, though: Once your craving is broken, you are less likely to relapse because you won't want to go through that distress again.

HABIT CATEGORY. Total your answers to F, L, and R. High scores indicate that you are a "reflex" smoker. For you, quitting may be relatively easy. Your goal is to break the link between smoking and your own triggering events—food, a cup of coffee, sitting down to work. Think of tapering off gradually. Each time you reach for a cigarette, stop and ask yourself *out loud*: "Do I really want this cigarette?" If you answer no, then skip it.

The higher your score in each category, the more that factor plays a role in your smoking. If you score low in all the categories, you probably aren't a long-term smoker. Congratulations—you have the best chance of getting off and staying off.

Combined high scores across several categories suggest that you get several kinds of rewards from smoking. For you, stopping may mean you need to try several different tactics. Being a high scorer in both *Tension* and *Addiction* is a particularly tough combination. You *can* quit—many such people have—but it may be more difficult for you than for others. If you score high in *Stimulation* and *Addiction*, however, you may benefit from changing your patterns of smoking as you cut down. Smoke less often, or only smoke each cigarette partway, inhale less, use tapering filters or low-tar/nicotine brands.

As Larry sat across from me in my office, I could sense the mixture of hope and skepticism on his face. He really wanted to quit, but the test indicated he was both addicted and used cigarettes for tension reduction. This helped explain why his quitting lasted only till the tension in his life built up again. I told him that he'd have to quit cold turkey and take up some form of yoga-like relaxation. Then I told him about the essential need for him to make an all-out commitment to end smoking forever.

Decision and Commitment

As I mentioned earlier, there are a number of techniques to help you quit smoking. The most important thing—the "key"—is the decision and the commitment. Then, having made the commitment, you can choose the technique that appeals most to you that is available. Here are a few.

DR. RYBACK'S TEN-STEP PROGRAM TO STOP SMOKING

1. Create a Supportive Environment

Get rid of all smoking paraphernalia from your home, office, and car—cigarettes, ashtrays, lighters. Let your friends and co-workers know in advance that you're quitting and solicit their support, so that they can offer you that rather than a cigarette, when the going gets rough. You'll find out who your real friends are.

2. Find a Buddy

A support group would be great, but that's not always available. If you can have a buddy quit with you, it's much less lonely. At least try and have a spouse, lover, or good friend be available as a full-time support. If all three are in one person, so much the better. If you know of someone who's quit in the past year or so, search that person out as a great source of understanding support.

3. Take Vitamin C

For the first week or so, put extra thought into having lots of fresh fruit and fruit juice. Make sure you're getting your share of vitamin C. This would be a good time to find out what your optimal dose is.

4. Exercise

It's also a good time to push yourself just a little bit on your exercise routine. Your first week of quitting is a good time to push the edges of the envelope just a little bit. Whatever you do, don't get into your couch-potato mode.

5. Give up Coffee—for a While

I hate to break this piece of news to you, but it would really help if you give up caffeine when you first give up smoking. I know this does-n't sound very appealing if you're a coffee drinker, but it's only temporary. You see, smokers process caffeine faster, and quitting smoking returns caffeine processing to normal. Since the caffeine stays in the ex-smoker's body longer than it used to, it creates a stronger case of the jitters—the last thing you need at this time. Also, you may have developed a strong habit of having a cigarette with your coffee—an extra temptation. So for those two good reasons, please forget about coffee and caffeinated soft drinks for a while.

6. Try Nicorette Gum and Skin Patches

According to a thorough review of the medical literature, the most successful approach to quitting smoking involves a combination of frequent face-to-face contact with a physician or psychologist or other professional who provides motivation and relevant information over the time period necessary to overcome the smoking habit, along with such prescription medications as Nicorette, the nicotine gum, or skin patches.

Nicorette may take a little getting used to. This gum is somewhat unfamiliar to taste, and there's a special method for chewing it which involves "parking" it in your cheek, then taking a few chews, "parking" again, and so on. But the great benefit is that you can give up your cigarettes immediately and wean yourself off the nicotine gradually. And this works!

Nicotine gum is the only proven drug treatment to help smokers quit. Nicorette, produced by Marion-Merrell Dow Pharmaceuticals of Kansas City, Missouri, is the only product of its kind currently in the U.S. Your physician must prescribe it. It does not cure the urge to smoke, but it does help you get through withdrawal and deal with irritability. In late 1991, prescribed nicotine came out in patch form under the brand names Nicoderm, Habitrol and ProStep. All you have to do is stick a patch on your upper arm and a trans-derm process releases nicotine through your skin gradually in tiny doses. These nicotine transdermal systems deliver nicotine through the skin in regulated doses in decreasing stages over time.

Speaking of patches, another aid to quitting is the drug Catapres (generically know as clonidine), whose primary function is to treat high blood pressure. But somehow, many have found a trans-derm patch of Catapres useful in overcoming the irritability and jitters associated with quitting smoking.

7. *Meditate* with Affirmations

Find a quiet place where you definitely will not be disturbed. For 15 minutes, before breakfast and before dinner, sit quietly and comfortably with your eyes gently closed and do the following three things:

a. Repeat the affirmation, "I enjoy looking younger and living longer in a smoke-free world."

b. As you do this, picture yourself looking youthful and radiant and feeling healthy and happy.

c. If any distracting thoughts or images come up, don't get disturbed. Merely accept them into your consciousness and then say a gentle "good-bye" to them as you return to your positive imaging and affirmation. With time, you'll learn to focus more clearly and have less distraction.

As time goes by, you may want to modify the affirmation to suit your own personality and needs. Please do so. Just make sure to continue this affirmation till you're clearly over the smoking habit.

8. Recognize the "Smoking Pangs" of Success

Remember the "hunger pangs of success," where hunger pangs are interpreted as signs of becoming a thinner person? See if you can do this with smoking urges. Label urges and irritability as signs of success, as reminders that you've conquered smoking. It's a bit more challenging than the hunger pangs technique, but see if it works for you.

9. Dealing with Urges

Whenever you have an urge to smoke, take a few minutes out to stand (if you're sitting), take a brief walk (around the office or outdoors), and help yourself to some deep breaths of air, blowing out slowly and forcefully. If you can, take a drink of cool water. Remember, the first three days are the roughest. It starts getting easier after that.

10. Become a Nonsmoker

Once you decide to quit and take action, you've become a nonsmoker. So choose the nonsmoking section in restaurants and airplanes. You're now going first-class, health-wise.

YOUR TASTE BUDS WAKE UP! One unpleasant item I've avoided till now is weight gain. Yes, chances are you may gain two to five pounds during this process. But although that's statistically true for most, it doesn't have to be for you. There are two major reasons you gain weight at this time. First, your taste buds and sense of smell are finally being liberated from the noxious effects of cigarette smoke. "Hallelujah!" they proclaim. "We had forgotten how good food can taste! How about some more of that linguine? And don't forget a little more of that acorn squash, while you're up. Just a smidgen of that butterscotch ice cream to top if off. Thanks."

ANY WEIGHT GAIN WILL BE TEMPORARY. The second reason you may gain weight is that your metabolism may slow down temporarily once you stop smoking. So for these two reasons, you'd be wise to emphasize fresh fruits and push your exercise a bit these first couple of weeks. Even if you do gain a bit of weight, you'll most likely lose it soon if you stick to the guidelines we've discussed all along.

WHY NONSMOKERS LOOK YOUNGER

First of all, it might be helpful to realize that in addition to the destructive effects of smoking mentioned thus far (carbon monoxide, cancer, atherosclerosis, and many other illnesses), there is one that directly affects your appearance. Smoking adversely affects circulation and as a result your skin gets less nourishment than it needs. Smokers tend to have less healthy, more wrinkled skin. By stopping smoking *now*, you can (depending on your current age) start adding one of the components of looking up to ten years younger.

In addition, those who are accustomed to smoking often have discolored fingers and nails, an unattractive characteristic which tends to add years to a man's apparent age.

On a less permanent basis, but even more offensive to many non-smokers, is the odor of smoke which attaches itself so readily to clothing and hair.

To this add cigarette breath, and you have a man who has lost his appeal to many otherwise interested partners. All in all, a man who doesn't smoke will more likely have a youthful, attractive effect on others than his counterpart who does smoke. So if you need more motivation to stop smoking, please be advised that you'll not only be physiologically younger, you'll also appear socially younger and more attractive as well.

HOW SMOKING CAN LEAD TO IMPOTENCE

Even worse than making you socially unattractive, smoking can definitely lead to impotence. Men who smoked one pack a day for five years were 15 percent more likely to suffer impotence, and men who smoked a pack a day for 20 years were 72 percent more likely to suffer impotence. The average age of these men? Only 35 years old! Smoking causes a significant narrowing of the artery to the penis in smokers. Furthermore, couples in which at least one member smokes are more than three times as likely to have trouble conceiving than nonsmoking couples.

All Patched Up and Ready to Go!

So here you are, ready to quit. A nicotine transdermal patch on one arm, a patch of Catapres on the other. You've tossed all smoking gear, and prepared your support systems. You can still vividly recall the sickening taste of that last cigarette you puffed on every 5 to 10 seconds.

The Whole Package: QUIT

In order to assist you in putting all this together, remember this QUIT package:

1. **Q**uestion why you smoke when you know clearly that smoking:
   ages your skin
   results in early death

2. **U**nderstand that quitting is a personal decision to:
   live longer
   look younger
   breathe easier
   kiss sweeter
   enjoy the flavors of food and the fragrances of flowers again

3. **I**nitiate:
   a support system
   a technology for quitting smoking, including patches
   an exercise program (if you haven't already)
   daily affirmations

4. **T**reat yourself to nonsmoking accommodations in:
   restaurants
   airplanes
   romantic relationships

Persistence! Easier the Next Time Around

If, despite all this, you somehow don't make it—it's okay! Don't give up. Get on the bandwagon again and go around one more revolution. You'll get through your *Denial* more quickly this time, as well as your *Conflict*. When you get to your *Action* phase, you will benefit from all you've learned the first time around. And your new *Change* mode will be even more effective.

Your Ultimate Success Is Guaranteed

But maybe I'm just blowing in the wind. Maybe you'll make it the first time around. If not, maybe the second, or third. But one thing is guaranteed. If you don't give up, you can surely quit eventually with persistence. It gets easier with time and experience. Looking years younger and living years longer is definitely worth the effort!

— SIDEBAR I —

SATIATION SMOKING

Satiation smoking consists of smoking your last cigarette with a vengeance. Having decided that this is your last cigarette, you make sure to inhale fully every 5 to 10 seconds until you've finished the cigarette. If you think that'd be fun, think again. You'll have to force yourself. You'll feel nauseated, dizzy, terrible. I don't recommend this for everyone. *Never* do it alone! Do it in the presence of your doctor. The idea is to give yourself such a sickening experience of smoking that you'll find it distasteful from then on.

— SIDEBAR II —

DR. DAVID RYBACK
CONTRACT TO QUIT SMOKING

I, _____, do hereby solemnly swear to quit smoking
                                          forever.
My quitting date will be _____.
    Between now and my quitting date, I will observe my smoking behavior, experiment with alternatives, record my urges and number of cigarettes smoked, and keep a smoking journal. During this time I will work daily to change my smoking-related thought patterns and to reduce my intake of tobacco smoke. On the day I have chosen, I will stop smoking forever.

_____   _____
        Name   Date

In witness whereof:

_____   _____
    Support Person   Date

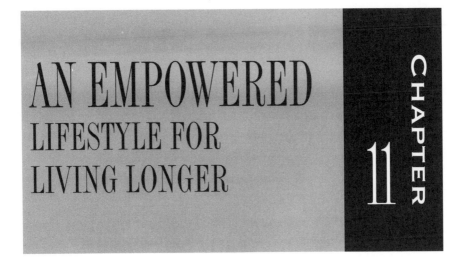

AN EMPOWERED
LIFESTYLE FOR
LIVING LONGER

CHAPTER
11

Over and over, we hear and read about scientific evidence that reducing stress makes for a stronger immune system and a longer, healthier life. In order to live ten years longer, it's essential to reduce stress in as many areas of personal experience as possible. In this chapter you'll learn ways to overcome personal problems and to live a longer, happier life by dealing with life's challenges directly and forthrightly and to use your added years of maturity to support others in living longer, healthier lives with less stress as well.

SEVEN SUGGESTIONS FOR BUILDING A STRONG SUPPORT NETWORK

This section is a review of some of the effective techniques mentioned earlier, brought together to form the basis of a rich, supportive personal network to be there through good times and bad. When problems do occur, you'll have friends to help you through them, so that stressful situations can be resolved quickly and effectively.

1. Be Helpful to Others So You Can Count on Them When You Need Help

Solid friendships are a two-way street. Only if both individuals are benefiting is the friendship strong enough to stand the test of time. The friendships you choose to foster can be maintained by ensuring that you offer at least as much as you get. For when you're in a pinch and needing your friend's help, it's unlikely that a promise to be a good friend from then on will do the trick. Only a history of mutual benefit will bear whatever strain your demands make at the time.

2. Have at Least One or Two Friends in Whom You Can Confide All Your Secrets without Reservation

By now you know the importance of having at least one or two such friends. The freedom to unburden your soul when you're particularly troubled by matters you can't share freely, for whatever reason, is priceless. Again, such trust can only be built on a history of confidentiality shared between you.

For most people, confidentiality is a joke. Typically, the best way to spread news of unusual behaviors or circumstances is to tell it to someone and add, "but this is confidential," and then in a hushed tone, "super confidential." You can bet dollars to doughnuts that the news will spread like wildfire, each person adding that urgent "super confidential" tag line that ensures the listener will rush to the next most intimate friend or lover and repeat the news, with slight distortion to add his or her own personal touch, again adding the tag line, "super confidential." It makes for a very efficient communication system.

The friends in whom you choose to confide are exceptions to this general rule. It may take years to build such trust and devotion, but the effort is well worthwhile. When the time comes, you'll have someone with whom to share your problems, and get a healthier perspective in all likelihood. In such fast friends, you have one of the most powerful of all stress-busters.

3. Don't Let Distance Be a Barrier—Use Letters, Fax, Phone, E-Mail to Communicate

One of the problems in nurturing such strong friendships is that you don't always have the good fortune of finding one in your immediate community. As your levels of responsibility and power grow, you're more and more likely to have opportunities for travel—to attend conventions, to meet clients, to offer seminars. You'll meet new friends and acquaintances and among these may be that special person you instinctively trust at some initial level. But he or she may live hundreds or even thousands of miles away. Usually that's enough to kill the possibility of a special friendship. But when it's not and you refuse to give up this opportunity, then you can easily overcome the distance between you by talking on the phone, sending faxes or, if you really want to be thoughtful with one another, good, old-fashioned letter writing. There's something about putting your feelings down on paper that's qualitatively different. It seems more personal and more permanent at one and the same time. So whatever form of communication you choose, you can easily overcome the distance between you and your special friend, especially if he or she is one of those special companions with whom you can open up without reservation, trusting implicitly in the bond of confidentiality between you.

4. Make It Your Business to Have Friends with the Expertise You May Occasionally Need

You alone are responsible for shaping the circle of friends you most desire. If you'd like this circle to be a resource of support to you in times of need, then the most direct way to assure this is to cultivate and foster such friendships. If you hesitate because of the fear that you might be using such relationships in a mercenary fashion, then think again about what I mentioned at the beginning of this section; any true friendship is based on mutual support. Think not what your friend can do for you, to paraphrase John Kennedy, think what you can do for your friend. Doctors, businessmen, lawyers, yes, and even plumbers, need friends too. What can you do for such friends? When you meet experts in fields of interest to you, and you genuinely like and trust these individuals, then reach out, ask some questions, and see if there's enough in common between you to invite friendship. And then think what you can do for your friend. It may be confidentiality, it may just be support offered during an occasional chat. But whatever it is, offer at least as much as you get.

5. Solve Your Problems on a Dependable, Routine Basis

Problems offer two options: one is worry, the other is solution. Many people procrastinate facing problems directly and choose to worry instead. That's a personal choice that you have in our free society.

The choice to solve your problems rather than to go on worrying about them is made easier by the rich network of support you can now build. Choose one particular time of the week to work on solving your problems. My particular time is Friday mornings.

Whatever problems come up in my life (and they do), I relegate to work on Friday mornings, no matter what part of the week such problems may arise—barring fire and flood, of course, or similar crises that demand immediate attention. I set aside a few hours then to size up the problem (I average about one or two a week) and decide on one of two possibilities: Can I solve the problem myself or, if not, whom can I contact who can either help me solve the problem directly or at least refer me to someone who can? I don't waste time burdening friends with my problems if they can't be of help in some way. (Of course, my special confidentiality friends hear of my problems any time we communicate, but these aren't the friends for Friday mornings, necessarily.)

In some cases, I may not call a friend at all, but rather an organization or agency that can provide me with special information. By waiting until Friday, I've had a chance to sleep on the problem, collect my thoughts (and anxieties sometimes) and focus sharply on constructive options.

If a particular medical symptom continues to bother me till Friday, I may then make an appointment with my doctor. If a legal concern or question haunts me, I may call a legal resource. If I feel I've hurt the feelings of someone important to me, I may reach out directly to correct that situation. If I'm on the verge of a risky investment, I may call a knowledgeable friend. If a professional matter concerns me, I may call either a colleague or one of the professional societies to which I belong. Whatever the matter, I focus on that particular resource that can be most helpful. That way, I avoid bothering my other friends with such problems and I can use our time together to be of support to them. I'll want their support when they can be of greatest help in the area of their particular expertise. Otherwise, I'm there for them.

Today, as I sit at my desk on a cloudy Friday afternoon in November, I can reflect on how I used this morning to solve some problems. My first meeting was with a lawyer friend who will be of enormous help in getting some documentation together for a presentation. We were able to sit in his living room over cups of hot tea, and catch up with one another before some good-natured brainstorming on how best to construct this presentation. (Of course, I paid him for his time. On the other hand, his rate was quite reasonable.)

Then off to my office to see some patients. I still had enough time left before lunch to make a few calls. I was concerned all week about the order of chapters for this book, so I called my editor, Douglas Corcoran, and suggested a change in sequence and offered the reasons for such a change. Doug said he'd think about it if I sent the suggested changes to him in writing.

Another concern that emerged during the week was the welfare of a couple of patients I hadn't seen in a while. Although I couldn't reach them by phone, I was able to leave messages for them so they could get back to me if they wished.

My final concern for the week was the need for letters of commendation to complete my application for acceptance in a professional organization. I made two calls—one to the president of an association, with whom I serve on the board, and one to the Chief Executive Office of the county where I live and for which I've offered free consulting as a civic volunteer. I knew I could count on both.

Now I can use the rest of the week doing constructive, fun things, refusing to waste my time worrying, until Friday morning when I gather my energies to focus on solutions once again.

6. Don't Waste Time on Individuals Who Drain You of Energy and Leave You Feeling the Worse for Wear

Of course, everyone has a right to be who he is, with all his unique characteristics. But some stand out as particularly draining. Occasionally, one such individual might be in a position to make demands for your attention even though you get annoyed and frustrated in this person's company. Even though you're adversely affected by this person, you might feel obligated to be available because of some special relationship—be it family, business-related or merely because this individual happens to be a friend of a friend.

Without being overly rejecting, you can best handle such a dilemma by discerning exactly what this person wants from you. It may be just your blind attention to their ongoing rambling. If so, try to match this person up with another lonely individual with much time on their hands so the two can form a satisfying relationship based on talking about whatever crosses their minds. Or that individual may be perseverating about some personal problem to which they respond "Yes, but . . ." to each valuable suggestion with which you come up—annoying, after a while.

In this case, give this individual your best shot at whatever advice you consider most useful and then, if that advice is ignored, just excuse yourself by saying: "I've got to go now, but let me know when you've had a chance to follow up on my suggestions and we'll take it from there. But since I'll be fairly tied up for a while, please wait until after you've tried my suggestions before you get back to me."

In either case, you take responsibility for the value of your own time and you've done what you can to respond to this individual's needs. If you allow your time to be consumed fruitlessly on ways that frustrate and annoy you, then there's no one to blame but yourself. By being direct and as helpful as you can in a concise but constructive way, you enrich this person all the more. And you free yourself up to spend your time more constructively, more enjoyably, and with less stress, to contribute to ten more healthy years.

7. Don't Resist Counseling or Psychotherapy When Any Problem Becomes Greater Than You or Your Network Can Resolve

Occasionally, despite your concerted efforts and the support of your friends, a problem may arise that persists, causing you an unusual degree of anxiety. If, after a few weeks, such anxiety persists, consider talking to a psychotherapist. Although expensive, such an individual is trained to listen attentively, consider all your lamentations, and help you reflect on your problem in such a way as to give you a liberating perspective.

In the end, the solution to your problem might be quite simple, but for some reason you've avoided it. That's probably why your friends' advice didn't help. You were blind to the obvious for some inner fear that you may have been harboring. A therapist's patient, sympathetic ear, and calm, reassuring manner will help you face that inner fear and overcome it constructively. So when friends and your own personal resources occasionally fall short in solving a deep problem, don't resist a professional's help. It's expensive, but a fall-back position you can't afford to be without on at least some occasions in your life.

PLAYING THE HAND THAT'S DEALT YOU

It always annoys me when I hear someone utter, after some unfortunate incident: "Well, things always work out for the best. There must be a reason for this (losing all one's money in an investment, having an expensive and painful accident, the death of a young friend) happening." It annoys me because such a statement preempts my feelings of anger or sadness. It also dismisses the significance of the event by attributing an anonymous, purposeless "meaning" to it. If there is meaning to it, then let that be my own discovery, coming from my own consideration of thoughts and feelings. In other words, don't tell me there's a meaning to it before I've had a chance to acknowledge my own feelings and then let the personally-felt meaning emerge naturally.

Don't dismiss personal failures out of hand by quickly saying: "Well, there must be a reason for that, but it's beyond me so I'll just go on with my life and pay no more mind to it."

Instead, find the opportunity for understanding, learning, and growth in each experience that is initially painful and punishing. Whatever hand is dealt you, play it to the optimum. That means, whatever setback befalls you, play it back in your mind until you can discover the specific elements of your involvement that led to the unhappy results. That way, you grow by becoming more mindful and aware when in similar circumstances in the future. It's called wisdom.

Even negative emotions, apart from accidents and mishaps, can be transformed into positive feelings when the same mindfulness is applied. For example, consider envy, a negative emotion by anyone's standard. By exploring this emotion closely, you can transform it into a highly enjoyable one. Envy is a feeling of being deprived of something you notice in someone else's life. If you can change your perspective and encourage yourself to enjoy this other person's satisfaction in a vicarious way, then you'll be able to feel a modicum of joy instead of the pain of deprivation. By enjoying his success vicariously, you can ultimately share in that experience of success. If your friend's success reminds you that you would like some of what he has, in addition to enjoying his success vicariously, find out (perhaps from him) what it takes, in terms of energy and focus, to acquire such success. You may even enlist your friend's support. Accept the hand that's dealt you, but if you choose a better hand, then you need to give up some cards from your own hand (time and energy), before you can pick up some unknown cards from the face-down deck (chance of success) to replace them. And whatever new cards you do pick up, play them as best you can, with confidence and optimism.

You determine your own success in many small, almost unnoticeable ways. Your life events can be predicted by your deeper expectations. Small and subtle behaviors accumulate to result in a decisive response, especially in social interactions. The more truly you expect something, the more your small and subtle expressions will result in the expected outcome. These small and subtle expressions communicate to others what's expected of them by you, and they typically oblige.

An obvious example of this: being stopped by a police officer for a traffic infraction. If you expect to be cited, the officer will happily oblige you. But if you truly feel innocent of the alleged infraction and your small and subtle expressions convey this, then the officer might just let you off with a warning. As a matter of fact, on a somewhat larger scale, that's what the legal jury system is all about. Six or twelve fellow citizens sit and watch the small and subtle expressions of the defendant and weigh these at least as heavily as the legal considerations of the case as they sort out their thoughts and feelings in the complex decision-making process. This is becoming more apparent as TV and print journalism analyze all the intricate components of the jury's decision-making process.

So by being increasingly aware of your true intentions and the subtle signals you convey to others, you can better play the hand that's dealt you. Go for what you want with what you have, directly and forthrightly. It's not a matter of luck. It's a matter of intention.

SIX STEPS TO UNDERSTANDING OTHERS AT A DEEPER LEVEL

Richard, a highly intelligent, successful businessman in his early 40s, was having trouble in his marriage. Whenever his wife suggested something to him, he'd describe his own position in such abstract terms and with such earnest zeal that her idea got totally transformed in the process. A look of frustrated puzzlement would appear on her face and she'd withdraw emotionally for a day or two. She'd been through this so many times without any success of communicating with Richard that resignation was all she had left.

After a long talk with Richard, I convinced him that his style of communication might be great at pushing decisions through committees but that it was destroying his marriage. Poor Richard looked at me in amazement. But he was intelligent enough to pick up on my suggestions very quickly once he realized he needed to change at home.

Communication takes place at two levels—one level is face value of the words spoken; the other is the intent, motivation, fears, and desires giving rise to the words expressed. By understanding the emotional origins of the words expressed, you're in the powerful position of cutting through such words to their deeper meaning.

You can know this deeper level not by any trick or gimmick, but by the genuine effort put into understanding the other's perspective as much as possible.

But first you need to learn to be sensitive to your own motivation, fears, and desires so that you have a clear channel through which to recognize the feelings of others. This is not accomplished overnight, but by a continuing process of facing the truth of your own experience with brutal honesty. "To thine own self be true," and honesty with others will follow naturally. Then you can read others more clearly and openheartedly.

The next skill to be learned is to become articulate in expressing your own feelings with honesty and to help others feel safe and fulfilled through your incisive awareness of their deeper strengths and vulnerabilities.

To enter into the inner world of the person you wish to understand more deeply, learn to put aside your own interests, at least temporarily. In this way, you can truly "walk in another's shoes."

The word "understand" can be seen as "standing under"—seeing the world from the other's unique, personal perspective. Only by forsaking your own perspective for the moment can you truly understand the other. Most people are unable to accomplish this. You can, if you devote yourself to the process. Here's how.

1. In your conversation, repeat what you've heard as if you had become the other. Pretend in your own mind that the other person has temporarily lost his or her ability to speak and you're doing your best to speak for him or her. Repeat what you've just heard as accurately as possible, repeating the exact words if possible, or paraphrasing as closely as you can. You can start off saying, "If I hear you right, you're saying that. . . ."

2. Having done this to the best of your ability, now check to see if there's accuracy in your perception. "Is that right?" or "Am I on target?" or "Do I understand what you're saying?"

3. You may be surprised to discover that you're off target a lot more than you expected, especially when you first start out. People think they hear more accurately than they typically do. Keep repeating steps 1 and 2 until you do get a response that you're close to being on target. Now you're ready for step number 3: Report the feeling or emotion you feel lies behind the other's statement, for example, "It feels as if you're angry (sad, hurt, ecstatic) about this," and follow up again with a check for accuracy, "Is that right?"

4. Always go with the other's corrections and forget about being right or wrong.

5. This is not about winning a debate, it's about getting close to the other so you can better understand him or her. As you continue in that process, be as openly supportive as you can in both manner and tone of voice. Maintain good eye contact and lean gently toward the other, with attentive interest. Avoid making any judgments about what you hear. Pretend you're inside the skin of the other, seeing things exactly the way he or she does.

6. Don't fear losing your own self, even though you're letting go of your own values and judgments temporarily. Your value system

will still be there after the conversation, and you'll actually become emotionally stronger in the process, with a somewhat more flexible, enlightened outlook on life. Having entered the perspective of another, your own perspective is now broadened.

As I continued my talks with Richard, he learned to use his quick mind to adopt this new, exciting form of communication with his wife. "I realize I've been in my own head all this time," he admitted. "I just never stopped to think about it this way before." After a while, Richard was using this new style of communication to overcome some problem relationships at work that had resisted his otherwise successful business style. Now Richard's marriage was like a second honeymoon and he was gaining a new kind of respect at work as well. His success both at home and at work was no longer hampered by his former inability to read other people.

As you foster this skill of understanding others better, including your mate, children, boss, and co-workers, you'll have considerably less stress in your life and you'll be adding another component to a longer, healthier life, not to mention greater happiness personally and more success professionally.

GOING WITH THE FLOW

Just as you can be sensitive to another's thoughts and feelings, so can you be sensitive to the changing and challenging events in your life. By giving up a rigid view of life and being open to the varied possibilities and their potential benefits, you can more easily adapt yourself to whatever challenges confront you.

Consider that there is no absolute truth. Certainly there are laws that, when broken and enforced, result in punishment. But at a more personal and philosophical level, the deepest truths are not easily captured in fixed rules. If there is one rule that leads to true happiness, it has more to do with genuineness and honesty than any other style or quality.

Any decision that can go either way—for instance, a dilemma— usually has no inherent correct answer. Either way is probably okay. By investing your ego one way, you may lose. By accepting either outcome as equally "right," you free yourself from attachment. Instead of deciding with your head, allow your heart to be open to both outcomes. Accept the one that emerges naturally as you support the welfare of others rather than your own selfish attachments.

A short time ago, I was to give a reading from a novel I'd written. The reading was to take place in a large auditorium. Concerned that so few people would attend that the audience would feel dwarfed by the large auditorium, a smaller room was reserved as an alternative. The day before the reading, however, a decision had to be made because of the time restrictions in setting up video cameras and lighting. I wanted the more professional lighting available only in the auditorium, so that the video would have a more professional look. On the other hand, the audience would, in all likelihood, feel more comfortable in the smaller room.

Overlooking my own selfish concerns, I intuitively chose the smaller room. When the time for the reading finally came, it became quite apparent I'd made the "right" choice, even taking my selfish concerns into consideration. What happened was that a technician-in-training had been assigned to run the camera. When my reading finally began, the individual in charge of the evening observed a pained look on the technician's face. Without hesitation, she rushed up to the technician and saw that she couldn't find the button that would start the recording. A couple of frantic phone calls later, and the problem was resolved.

When I discovered this at the end of my reading, after a few moments of anger and disappointment, I realized that the whole problem could have been resolved by recording the first ten minutes of the reading (the part originally missed) over again, even though the audience had already gone. This was simple enough to do. After editing, the end result might even be better.

Now, had I chosen the more selfish alternative to read in the larger, but darker auditorium, the person in charge would never have been able to see the look of desperation on the face of the shy technician. The whole reading would have transpired without the correct record button ever having been found. And my hoped-for tape would never have been made. Moral? When faced with a dilemma, you never really know which choice is better. If the pull to either side is about the same, choose the one that benefits others as well as yourself. Chances are it'll come out better for you as well.

RISING ABOVE THE FURY: FOUR STEPS TO CONQUERING STRESS AND ANXIETY DUE TO MAJOR CRISES

Despite the best of intentions and the most open of hearts, occasionally life deals a devastating blow. Whatever the nature of the threat, or loss, the adrenaline flows, sleep is lost, and anxiety pervades. What to do to cope with such threats?

1. Imagine the worst possible outcome and the consequences of that. If that worst outcome is death, then you can surrender yourself to the profession and technology of medicine and accept such support. If that outcome is financial ruin, then consider how you would accept a different level of material consumption. If that outcome is legal prosecution, then consider how justice prevails, and accept your punishment or assert your innocence. In most cases by far, the outcome is not so severe, but by considering the worst, you can more easily deal with the rest.

2. Solicit the support of the most capable professionals available to you—doctors, lawyers, financial experts. Give in to their expertise.

3. Realize the ultimate rule of overwhelming problems: This too shall pass! At least you have a chance. You can't lose anything by banking on that chance.

4. Having done all this, accept anxiety as just another experience of life. And watch it disappear.

HEALTHY PROBLEM-SOLVING WITH A HEALTHY BODY

In Chapter Seven, I focused on how to initiate and maintain an effective fitness program.

One factor outweighs all others in acquiring and maintaining a healthy body: a desire to participate in and enjoy disciplined physical activity that is challenging and satisfying. The key is to enjoy such activity and to experience a sense of fulfillment as one goes from level to level of challenge.

A fit and healthy body makes all challenges somewhat more approachable. With more vigor and energy, intellectual, administrative, and creative efforts are more easily tackled. In addition, being fit contributes to a greater sense of self-esteem.

A moderate, ongoing involvement in an enjoyable activity can cost little effort, once the routine is well-established. For those men who enjoy challenge or competition, fitness activities such as team sports and footraces provide these. A brisk walk is excellent for those men who don't take to intense activity.

The key is to develop an appetite for such physical activity, if it isn't yet developed. Once fitness becomes part of your life, and you experience the stamina, energy, and confidence as a result, you're a step ahead in terms of solving your personal problems.

SHARPENING YOUR INTUITION TO HELP YOU MAKE BETTER DECISIONS

To begin with, intuition and gut feelings are typically more reliable and trustworthy in the long run than what your brain can tell you. Your brain works with all the data you're aware of. Your intuition includes all these data and then some, such as data you have in your brain, but that you can't articulate in thoughts or words. These subconscious data are at the feeling level.

You can't remember everything you see and hear, but all data that enter your brain through your senses are virtually trapped there till you die. You can only put into words or conceptualize a tiny fraction of all the data trapped within your skull. The part that you can put into words is what psychologists refer to as conscious mind. All the rest—the data that can't be expressed in words because they haven't been processed by certain components of the "thinking" cerebral cortex—is called the *unconscious*.

When you decide with your thoughts alone, you're using only a small fraction of all your brain data. When you use your intuition to help you decide, you're able to use more data that you can't put into words, yet you can still sense through your bodily feelings. This is what women refer to as "intuition" and what men call "a gut feeling." Since intuition uses bodily feelings as well as conceptual data, more data is available, therefore resulting in a better or "smarter" judgment or decision.

In order to foster such intuition and "inner wisdom," begin by taking some time each day to meditate in a comfortable setting, free from distraction, and free from any attempts at problem solving. See Chapter Three on stress reduction for specific details. In this way, you can begin to tune in to all those data that are not otherwise available and feed them into the decision-making process. You can then expect to make sounder decisions and wiser judgments.

MINIMIZING PERSONAL CONFLICT BY EXPRESSING GRATITUDE

Expressing gratitude is a simple yet very effective habit for making all your relationships run much more smoothly. In this way, you can strengthen the sources of support that enrich your life. You can consolidate that positive stream of giving that makes you feel more secure and fulfilled. Start with those closest to you. The closer the relationship, the more warmly expressed the gratitude.

There are many overlooked possibilities for expressing gratitude within your own family. When your mate helps you with the dishes, office work, or other chores, does she feel taken for granted? She won't if you make a habit of thanking her. What about your children? Do you think they'd be more likely to clean up their rooms or take out the garbage if you remembered to thank them on a consistent basis? Personal conflicts within your family might be reduced considerably by these simple measures.

This works with co-workers, as well. If you remember to thank them for the little acts of assistance and consideration that come your way, then these helpful acts will only increase and endure.

Thanking your subordinates for fulfilling their duties is nothing less than good management.

What about gratitude expressed to your superiors? Sound odd? An occasional brief note, sincerely expressed, and sincerely felt, expressing appreciation for a policy decision you truly support, can let them know that you're comfortable being a team player. Of course, if you're at all oversolicitous in your tone, this can come across as brown-nosing. But if you can express your gratitude concisely and with a professional tone, then such communications can only do you good.

If your life is going fairly well, and you do appreciate that it is, a general attitude of gratitude can be expressed by small and large acts of generosity to those not yet in your support network, in other words, to life as a whole. This expression can extend toward those you serve in your job, career, or profession. This attitude can only enhance your relationship with those you serve and make your life work more meaningful and enjoyable.

Reducing interpersonal conflict comes from your attitudes and actions, by performing deeds and saying things that contribute to richer, more meaningful relationships, to a greater sense of self-esteem and ultimately to a fulfilling sense of purpose or mission.

The more you can acquire the habit of expressing gratitude, through appreciating and supporting others, the happier you'll feel, and the healthier your mental state and physical health.

BECOMING A BETTER PROBLEM SOLVER BY BECOMING A VOLUNTEER

As an extension to acquiring the habit of expressing gratitude, you have the opportunity to contribute aspects of your energy and talents to organizations, be they health-care agencies, professional organizations, educational institutions, or political parties. You can volunteer to help the sick or needy, to support the organizations that represent your job or profession, to teach or coach some inner talent you enjoy sharing, or to support the candidacy of politicians who express your values.

Despite my busy lifestyle, I'm committed to offering my services as a voluntary contribution to at least one or more organizations. In the past, I've been a speaker for the American Cancer Society, a national cancer organization, and other health-oriented societies. I've done counseling at a local church. More recently, I've donated my time as an organizational consultant to the government of the county in which I live. This activity has not only given me the opportunity to meet a number of interesting and effective administrators, but also put me in touch with sources of support that I might need at some time in my life. Beyond that, I enjoy a sense of civic pride, knowing that I can be a helpful part of my local government. You can do this too, without waiting to be appointed or going through a campaign for election. Just offer the best talents you have and the skills you've acquired. There's always room for a good and effective volunteer.

Any of these volunteer activities will help you become a better problem solver and minimize personal problems in the following ways:

1. You'll have the opportunity to meet interesting, influential, and typically supportive individuals who can be models for you to become a better problem solver. These successful individuals can also be models for dealing with life's problems by avoiding them through foresight and appropriate preventive measures.

2. You'll have an opportunity to explore your hidden potential—resources and talents heretofore undeveloped. The demands made on you may be very different from those with which you're familiar in your regular work, releasing a side of you that would otherwise remain untapped.

3. You'll gain more experiences in assuming responsibilities that are new for you and in coordinating your talents with those of others. Such new talents and coordinating skills will definitely make you more efficient at solving problems and paving the way for smooth personal relationships.

4. By interacting with people with diverse lifestyles and different perspectives, you'll broaden your own perspective and become more understanding of other points of view. This broader perspective will make you a better problem solver and minimize conflicts due to differing viewpoints.

This habit of contributing to social, professional, and political organizations should be fostered until it becomes strongly ingrained. As personal problems and interpersonal conflict become more easily resolved, you'll feel happier and more fulfilled.

By following the suggestions and examples I've offered in this chapter, you can not only get rid of personal problems as they occur and prevent many from occurring in the first place; you can also look forward to living a life of dignity and fulfillment, enjoying richer and deeper relationships with those at home and at work—a life of the highest quality, given your circumstances. Appreciate the uniqueness of every individual you come across; stay in touch with special friends, no matter where they live; listen with your heart as well as your head; and know when to lean on others. When your cup fills to the brim, give some back in terms of appreciation, gratitude, and some form of service to your community. You'll get it back, in spades. And a life of more joy and less stress will help you live ten years longer as well.

— CHART I —
PROBLEM-FREE LIFESTYLE

Problem:	Solution:
Need for support when you're feeling alone and isolated?	Nurture friendships with those who are helpful and supportive.
No one around to share with?	Get with the electronic age—use the phone, mail, e-mail.
Worry-wart?	Limit worrying to $1/2$ hour per day or one morning per week, to solve problems.
Feeling foolish for making an extremely poor judgment call?	Analyze the details and learn from your errors.
Pattern of repeated failures?	Learn to anticipate success by welcoming it in your moment-to-moment life experiences.
Realizing a pattern of making wrong choices?	Give up your selfish viewpoint and let your intuition guide you.
Feeling stressed and anxious about a possible crisis?	Imagine the worst, work for the best, and realize that ultimately this too shall pass.

Feeling misunderstood and unappreciated?	Learn to enter the "feeling-world" of others.
Feeling envious of another's success?	Learn to enjoy your friend's success vicariously.
Feeling old and worn out?	Get physical.
Feeling empty with loved ones and co-workers?	Communicate gratitude for what matters to you at every opportunity.
Feeling guilty about having so much success?	Share your resources: teach, coach, write, volunteer.

I've done my best to provide you with the most useful and practical information to help keep you living ten years longer and looking ten years younger. But additional information keeps coming up as research continues on this most vital subject. In order for you to stay abreast of the latest news and information on this topic, I've initiated a monthly information update to keep you at the cutting edge with the least effort on your part. A free sample of the *Live Longer Newsletter* is available at the following address:

Dr. David Ryback
1534 N. Decatur Road
Atlanta, Georgia 30307

I hope to hear from you.

INDEX